Routledge Revivals

Philosophy, Psychiatry and Psychopathy

First published in 2000, *Philosophy, Psychiatry and Psychopathy* was highly topical in tackling the interface of applied philosophy and psychiatry at a time when government and clinicians were giving careful consideration to new forms of treatment for people with psychopathic disorder.

The book brings together contributions from lawyers, philosophers, psychiatrists and clinical managers to explore the inter-related conceptual and political implications of Psychopathy.

Philosophy, Psychiatry and Psychopathy will appeal to those with an interest in the history and development of theories and research relating to philosophy and psychiatry.

Philosophy, Psychiatry and Psychopathy

Personal Identity in Mental Disorder

Edited by Christopher Heginbotham

Routledge
Taylor & Francis Group
ROUTLEDGE REVIVALS

First published in 2000
by Ashgate

This edition first published in 2021 by Routledge
2 Park Square, Milton Park, Abingdon, Oxon, OX14 4RN
and by Routledge
711 Third Avenue, New York, NY 10017

Routledge is an imprint of the Taylor & Francis Group, an informa business

Publisher's Note
The publisher has gone to great lengths to ensure the quality of this reprint but points out that some imperfections in the original copies may be apparent.

Disclaimer
The publisher has made every effort to trace copyright holders and welcomes correspondence from those they have been unable to contact.
These are re-issues of books published some years ago which are inevitably a reflection of the time in which they were published. The language used is indicative of that time and as such no offence is intended by the re-issuing of the books. The content is likewise reflective of the original year of publication.

A Library of Congress record exists under LCCN: 99085921

ISBN 13: 978-1-138-72199-9 (hbk)
ISBN 13: 978-1-315-19390-8 (ebk)
ISBN 13: 978-1-138-72196-8 (pbk)

DOI: 10.4324/9781315193908

Philosophy, Psychiatry and Psychopathy

Personal identity in mental disorder

Edited by
CHRISTOPHER HEGINBOTHAM

Ashgate

Aldershot • Burlington USA • Singapore • Sydney

Published by
Ashgate Publishing Ltd
Gower House
Croft Road
Aldershot
Hants GU11 3HR
England

Ashgate Publishing Company
131 Main Street
Burlington
Vermont 05401
USA

Ashgate website: http://www.ashgate.com

British Library Cataloguing in Publication Data
Philosophy, psychiatry and psychopathy : personal identity in mental disorder
1. Mentally ill - Psychology 2. Personality - Philosophy
3. Psychotherapy 4. Mental health - Philosophy
I. Heginbotham, Christopher II. Society for Applied Philosophy
155.2'0874

Library of Congress Control Number: 99-85921

ISBN 1 84014 864 0

Printed and bound by Athenaeum Press, Ltd., Gateshead, Tyne & Wear.

Contents

List of Contributors

Dr. Gwen Adshead, Consultant Psychiatrist and Hon Senior Lecturer, St. George's Hospital, London and Broadmoor Hospital, Berkshire

Dr. Piers Benn, Lecturer in Philosophy, Imperial College, University of London

Prof. K.W.M. (Bill) Fulford, Professor of Philosophy and Mental Health, University of Warwick, Coventry

Christopher Heginbotham, Chief Executive, East & North Hertfordshire Health Authority, Welwyn Garden City

Prof. R.D.(Bob) Hinshelwood, Professor of Psychoanalysis, Centre for Psychoanalytic Studies, University of Essex, Colchester

Dr. Jeremy Holmes, Consultant Psychiatrist and Psychotherapist, North Devon Healthcare NHS Trust, Barnstaple

Martin Johnston, Department of Health Studies, University of Central Lancashire, Preston

Dr. Stephen Wilkinson, Department of Philosophy, Keele University, Staffordshire

1 Philosophy, Psychiatry and Personal Identity

Clinics, Concepts and Philosophy of Psychopathy

CHRISTOPHER HEGINBOTHAM

This book arose out of a conference organised by the Society for Applied Philosophy in 1997 to explore conceptual issues at the interface of philosophy, psychiatry, psycho-analysis, and law. Conference participants brought a wealth of experience and insights across the whole field of mental disorder, but the main elements of participants' papers and the ensuing discussion focused on the problems of personal identity and disordered personality, with specific attention to psychopathic personality disorder. A number of the papers collected here deal with the construction of personal identity and identification, but the depth of analysis of personality disorder at the conference was somewhat unexpected, and suggested that the focus of this book should be on psychopathy.

Psychopathic personality disorder (sometimes called psychopathy, or severe personality disorder, or sociopathy) is a clinical and social presentation which has challenged philosophers, psychiatrists, psychologists and lawyers for many years. There is no single definition of psychopathy nor a common understanding of the aetiology, taxonomy and genealogy of psychopathy. Working criteria have been established (Hare, 1980) and an expanding literature testifies to the burgeoning interest in psychopathic personality disorder. One reason why psychopathy has been under-researched is that for many years medicine (psychiatry) has considered persons with psychopathy to be untreatable and therefore to be outside the normal realm of psychiatric intervention. The 1980s and 1990s, however, have witnessed significant progress in the development of psychological therapies, notably but not exclusively cognitive behaviour therapy and forensic psychotherapy, and these clinical interventions have begun to demonstrate real success in the treatment of conditions hitherto considered refractory.

The emergence of therapeutic modalities relevant to psychopathic personality disorder (PPD) has occurred in parallel with at least two other important developments. The first is an increasing concern amongst politicians and the general public about mentally disordered offenders, many of whom are perceived to have some form of 'untreatable' mental health problem. During the 1990s in the UK alone there have been over 50 major inquiries (either sitting or finalised) into homicides by mentally disordered people, many of which have identified offenders as having some form of psychopathic or sociopathic disorder. The disorders presenting in these cases were perceived to be of such a nature and degree that the statutory psychiatric services were unable or unwilling to provide treatment. The Mental Health Act 1983 (England and Wales) - and associated Acts for Scotland and Northern Ireland - allows the civil detention of people with mental disorder only when there is some form of 'medical' treatment available for the disorder. The courts have steadily widened the meaning of the terms 'medical' and 'treatment' to include a wide range of medical, psychological and nursing treatment and care, but there remains a strong prejudice within psychiatry that PPD is untreatable.

Acceptance of the un-treatability of PPD has a long history, but the screw was tightened further by the 1970s debate on treatability as a test for compulsory admission to hospital. Publications such as 'A Human Condition' (Gostin 1975) took a human rights perspective in proposing that no person should be detained involuntarily unless there was a treatment available for his or her condition. The subsequent 20 years have seen a steady change in attitudes towards treatability, partly as a result of the emergence of new therapies, partly as a reaction to homicides and other serious incidents perpetrated by people with mental disorder, and partly from the recognition that there is a spectrum of behaviour and disorder and that a few patients are 'truly refractory'. Developments in forensic psychotherapy, the work of the Portman Clinic with sex offenders, pioneering work with violent prisoners, and the work of therapeutic communities such as the Cassel Hospital and the Henderson Clinic, are just a few examples which point to the relevance of providing therapeutic opportunities for such individuals.

Overcoming the deep seated prejudice against treatment for people with PPD has been a long and up hill struggle. The gradual acceptance of psychotherapeutic understanding and techniques has been one element of these changing attitudes. Another has been the recognition of the damaging effects of childhood physical and sexual abuse. Pioneering and innovative work such as de Zulueta's 'From Pain to Violence' (1993) have begun to change the perception of many clinicians to the therapeutic possibilities which might be available. A recognition and an understanding of the developmental processes which lead to PPD are a first step in developing intervention strategies as well as providing a focus on primary, secondary and tertiary prevention.

We should not assume, however, that PPD is a single disorder with a straightforward aetiology. Not only does the extent of the disorder, as manifest through antisocial behaviour, fall on a long spectrum from 'normal' social behaviour to that which is wholly aberrant, but there may be, as with many other mental disorders, a number of different disease entities bound up in present ways of describing PPD. Defining the various elements of PPD is a complex and demanding task. One approach to showing the difference between PPD and other forms of deviance is to consider offending behaviour by paedophiles, which is distinct from but often confused with the behaviour of those with PPD. Paedophilia is an example which may suffice to demonstrate a first step in unpicking the complex aetiology and presentation often conflated as PPD.

Paedophilia is perceived understandably by the majority of members of society as a severely aberrant, unattractive and unwanted form of perssonality The 'folk' perception of paedophilia has a number of intertwining strands. These comprise, as a minimum, (a) that paedophiles are dangerous criminals whose behaviour must be stopped more or less at any cost; (b) that if such people cannot see the error of their ways they are either mad, or bad, or both, and (c) in any event custodial care should be provided to ensure that they cannot re-offend. If we analyse the nature of sex offending, especially paedophilia, we can see some very significant differences from those features which we find in PPD (Carson and Heginbotham, Chapter 9).

It turns out in practice that the distinction between PPD and paedophilia is simple and clear cut. More challenging is the possible distinction between primary and secondary psychopathy (Mealey 1997) and whether a primary and secondary characteristics sometimes are combined in the single individual. Similarly Blair (1998) has suggested that individuals with aggressive antisocial tendencies tend to come from environments in which violence against others is a way of acquiring status. If the individual has an emotional deficit that tends to psychopathy, then his or her behaviour is likely to be particularly dangerous. In Blair's view, the person will lack a mechanism that would tend to inhibit antisocial behaviour in other people. Blair proposed (1993) a model for the development of morality which implies a specific cause for psychopathy. He suggested that in individuals whose behaviour is socially responsible there may be a 'violence inhibition mechanism' (VIM), a cognitive mechanism which is activated by non-verbal signs of distress and initiates a withdrawal response. Psychopaths lack this VIM and thus the distress cues which reduce aggressive behaviour in the majority of individuals cause no affect in those with psychopathic disorder.

The papers collected in this publication seek to address some of these challenging issues. The interest of contributors is in the clinical and philosophical manifestations of psychopathy as a mental disorder, rather than in psychopathy as a sociopathic trait. It has been suggested that in it's sociopathic manifestation, psychopathic tendencies, if intelligently used by their 'owner', may be of great value in business or commerce (Mealey 1997). Primary psychopaths act intentionally in an antisocial manner having reached a certain level of cognitive development at which they are able to distinguish emotions of the self from the emotions of others. On this basis, primary psychopaths are not incapable of empathy with others but rather choose intentionally not to empathise. This suggests a 'bad' rather than 'mad' model of behaviour.

On this argument, highly successful business people demonstrate at least an element of sociopathy; they are able to understand the effect of what they are doing on others but at the same time discount the moral or psychological harm that they are causing. From a game-theoretic perspective a small percentage of such individuals in society will be highly successful. Once the proportion reaches some index level, however, such individuals will begin meeting similar individuals too frequently, and, on average, their success rate will diminish. The evolutionary dynamics of primary psychopathy suggests that sociopathic behaviour will be stable whilst the numbers remain small.

Secondary psychopathy on the other hand describes those people whose development has been affected as a result of environment, nurture or abuse (or some other factor) and are unable to form appropriately empathetic relations with others. The development of an individual's desire to engage in acceptable and normative behaviour appears to be reasonably consistent from an early age. There are however differing theories of moral development. Kohlberg (1964) suggested that moral development advances in parallel with reasoning ability and thus differences in moral understanding can be attributed to differences of intellectual or cognitive ability. Conversely, Blair (1995) suggests that amongst other elements of psychological structure, there is the 'violence inhibition mechanism' (discussed above) and this must be initiated or primed before the individual can achieve full moral development. Lack of this mechanism is crucial to the establishment of psychopathic disorder. Alternatively the 'violence inhibition mechanism' may not be developed adequately; and it is possible that cognitive abilities are impaired also leading to impaired moral reasoning.

An alternative approach to the aetiology of secondary psychopathy is provided by, amongst others, de Zulueta (1993), drawing heavily on psycho-analytic theory to describe the effects of childhood physical, sexual or psychological abuse. There may be a number of ways in which such abuse leads to psychopathic personality. From a Kleinian perspective it will lead the individual to identify him or herself with a bad object leading to damage or destruction of self esteem and thus to an undermining of empathy with others.

The difference between primary and secondary psychopathy may be explained in differences in developmental environment. If there is a violence inhibition mechanism (which we might suppose can be more or less active) it suggests that some people have an emotional deficit but are not nurtured in an environment which triggers overly aggressive behaviour. We might speculate that some of those people will channel their emotional deficit into higher status activities - such as aggressive business practices - and develop behaviours which are psychologically rather than physically violent. If this is true then a further difference emerges.

As we have seen, evolutionary dynamics (Colman and Wilson 1997) suggest that some small proportion of persons with psychopathy in the community is an evolutionary stable position, and will settle down at some small percentage of the population, typically to 2-4%. Evolutionary dynamics using game theory based on the well known 'chicken' (or hawk/dove) game provides a mechanism for determining the equilibrium level. A higher percentage and each person with psychopathic tendencies will meet other similar individuals too frequently; much less than 2% and there will be 'opportunities' for antisocial gain which are not taken up!

This theory also suggests that, for secondary psychopaths particularly, the relative gain for the antisocial person is much less than the potential loss to the other person in any interaction. The example given by Colman and Wilson is that a mugger may gain only a small amount from assaulting or even killing a passer-by, but that the consequences for the victim may be catastrophic. This might not be true however for the person who operates in a sophisticated and psychologically aggressive fashion. In this case the gain may be very significant at the expense of relatively low losses to many people - for example small shareholders on the stock exchange. There may thus be two quite different forms of psychopathy in practice although linked causally dependent on the level of deprivation in childhood and the extent to which this damages the violence inhibition mechanism (if such a mechanism exists).

A key element in any discussion of PPD is the notion of empathy. By empathy we mean the ability of individuals to understand the effect of their own actions on others. Empathy has been defined as 'an affective response more appropriate to someone else's situation than to ones own' (Hoffman, 1987, p48). It is often assumed, perhaps wrongly, that having empathy or being able to empathise with others leads individuals to treat others as they would wish to be treated. As George Bernard Shaw once remarked - you "do not treat others as you would want to be treated, their tastes may not be the same". Paradoxically primary psychopaths may be able to empathise, in the sense of understanding the affective response of the other person, but not feel that affective response personally.

We may have to accept either (a) that some persons with PPD have empathy as defined but are able to use that empathy self interestedly knowing that the other person will be harmed in some way; or (b) our definition of empathy must be enhanced to emphasise not only the 'affective response' but to incorporate the idea that the person acts appropriately and normatively as a result of that affective response. In other words empathy is more than "an emotional response [or emotional reaction] to a representation of another's internal state",.... but incorporates an intention to act normatively in response to that emotional state. Psychopathic 'empathy' may be only partial or limited empathy such that the person understands the internal state of emotion generated in the other person but does not in turn have a fully developed emotional response to the other's state.

Exploration of empathy is a crucial element to understanding PPD. In Chapter 2 Gwen Adshead describes the notion of empathy as affective resonance and the ability vicariously to introspect. She explores whether empathy can be dismantled and how empathy is acquired and developed in children. Attachment theory and failure of attachment and of parenting suggests that the establishment of empathy is a necessary factor in achieving 'selfhood'. Empathy is also defined by Piers Benn in Chapter 3 in Strawson's terms as 'participant reactive attitudes'. PPD leads us to suspend participant attitudes under certain circumstances because we perceive psychopaths as lacking effective participant attention and are thus excluded from a rational web of public attitudes. But this leads to a further paradox. If persons with psychopathy have no moral sensitivity then surely society has the right to treat such people as outside the normal web of participant involvement and to be excluded and shut out of society completely. Yet we cannot say such persons are non-human, for they evidently are humans; but they appear to lack some element of what it means to be 'truly' or 'fully' human, in the sense of being an authentic and integrated member of the human community.

Primary psychopaths on the definitions provided here are bad, not mad, and are callously indifferent to the hurt of others even though they may understand what that hurt is. When the hurts and harms generated by such psychopaths reach some threshold of societal tolerance, society then has the right to exclude that person completely from social discourse. Conversely secondary psychopaths could be considered truly mentally ill - they have a mental disorder as a result of mental conditioning and are thus worthy of society's care and concern. Secondary psychopaths are 'genuinely', authentically mad, (or at least, mentally 'damaged') unable to empathise, perhaps as a result of dysfunctional nurture, and thus have a right to all the resources that society can provide to enable them to overcome the disorder from which they are suffering.

Although Strawson's concept of 'participant reactive attitudes' is helpful in widening our understanding of empathy, it may be insufficient or inappropriate in explaining the lack of prudential judgement in persons with secondary psychopathy. Primary psychopaths appear to have reasonably well developed cognitive abilities to make complex judgements about the reactions of others whilst discounting the hurt felt by others. Secondary psychopaths, on the other hand, whilst making good 'street wise' judgements of immediate necessity, are usually bad at making longer term judgements of their own best interests (Maher, 1990). On the Strawsonian view, moral responsibility need not imply the actual application of reactive attitudes. It only requires that the person be a candidate for such attitudes. It is thus essential to consider what participant reactive responses are generated in the person and the extent to which an individual is reactive and responsive to reasons.

It has been suggested recently that for an individual to be morally responsible for an action the person must have a mechanism that is reasons-responsive. (Fischer and Ravizza 1998). Such 'reasons-responsiveness' requires both an internalist and externalist conception of moral responsibility rather than the traditional exclusively internalist conception. There are two elements to this. First, the arrangement of an individual's mental states and how that arrangement developed are both important. In other words, the person's reactive attitudes need to be considered in the context of the development of such attitudes especially for those with secondary psychopathy. Second, the person's relationship to the real world is an essential component of moral responsibility. Fischer and Ravizza argue that appropriate reasons - responsiveness is a necessary condition for moral responsibility. 'We look for certain patterns of reasons - recognition, a kind of sensitivity to external reality, as well as minimal reactivity to reasons' (pp. 252, 253).

An integration of internalist and externalist approaches to moral responsibility has both clinical and philosophical implications. Clinically it provides a rationale for psychological therapies which seek to change the development of mental state arrangements; philosophically we can see a way to achieving a compatibility between moral responsibility and causal determinism. Moral responsibility and reasons-responsiveness may be straightforwardly consistent with certain forms of indeterminism. We cannot reject internal causes for 'mental disorder' but nonetheless must challenge or reject exclusively internalist claims and develop a richer conception of the development and application of morally responsible attitudes.

In Chapter 4, Bill Fulford considers some of the philosophical issues that have been raised by cross-disciplinary work between philosophy and psychiatry. He contends that we must be concerned with the 'real' person, not just with the brain alone, or just with the mind alone. This holistic approach challenges the dualism inherent in seeing a person and her mental disorder as distinct and separate elements. Although the case study Fulford uses is concerned with personality change, the implications for personal identity and especially psychopathy are readily apparent. Psychopathic personalities should not be treated as somehow 'fragmented' between the 'bad' (voluntarily breaching social norms) or the 'mad' (unable to recognise or act on social norms). By implication this challenges the idea of untreatability, by suggesting that a new paradigm of integration is needed.

Similarly, Martin Johnston, in Chapter 5, contrasts two approaches to mental illness - the 'realist' model, and the Szaszian or 'mythical' model. He concludes that manifestations of mental illnesses, such as delusions and hallucinations, are not arbitrary constructions, but are central to the identity of the person. The only myth is that disabling facets of mental illness are simply social constructs grafted onto an otherwise 'whole' person; in that sense Johnston also challenges the fragmentary or dualistic approach to mental disorder, and the notion that an 'illness' response requires an underlying disease entity as a sustaining cause.

An example of an affective response continuing in the absence of a distinct sustaining cause is provided by Stephen Wilkinson, in Chapter 6. He explores the nature of grief. Grief is usually a healthy reaction to distress but may become unhealthy if it continues for too long. However, grief has a continuing effect and could be considered a 'malady' even in the absence of a distinct sustaining cause. A person is often considered to be mentally disordered when abnormal responses continue in the absence of sustaining causes. Psychopathy is no exception to this argument. An acute or short lived lack of empathy for others may result from an accident, stress or personal tragedy. Usually the persons demeanour returns to its normative state once the initial cause is over. But this is not true in psychopathy where abnormal affect continues and in itself becomes normative. As Wilkinson shows however there are socially acceptable examples of affective responses continuing in the absence of a distinct sustaining cause. Although grief is the paradigm example demonstrating a continuing affective response without an obvious disease entity, even grief can become pathological if it continues for more than one to two years.

The following chapters explore further the idea of integration and personal identity from a psychodynamic perspective. Jeremy Holmes in Chapter 7 argues for an integration of the three models of mental disorder most often used - the biological, the social, and the dynamic. He suggests that overlaps and interplays between models are becoming more common, but that medical and social models require a 'psychodynamics' in order to achieve a fully informed perspective. The key determinants of the outcomes of any situation - loss, change, distress, threat- rest on the dynamics of personal development. Only a narrative biography - the stories that individuals tell about themselves - will provide the basis for a full understanding of the individual response.

Bob Hinshelwood argues in a similar vein in Chapter 8, but takes an institutional perspective as a way of exploring personal identity. Persons do not exist in isolation - by implication the development of personality disorder is dependent on interaction with other persons - and personal identity is formed from a process of identification of the self in relation to others. This process is conducted within an interpersonal medium and must be distinguished from the experience of identity. Paradoxically, there appears to be a genuine discontinuity within individuals, and a continuity between individuals.

Finally in Chapter 9, Chris Heginbotham explore another form of institutional response - that of law. Recent advances in therapeutic jurisprudence have recognised the value of tailoring legal formulation to the therapeutic objectives of society and of those charged with providing treatment and care for disordered individuals. Understanding personal identity is crucial to an effective jurisprudential response, especially in relation to psychopathy, as that response turns resolutely on the notion of treatability. If identity is in some sense fixed, and the person is not able to react participatively to others, then the legal response will be communitarian; if the person is able to some degree to reflect and to pursue a process of interpersonal identification, then the legal framework should provide that opportunity, however long that might take.

References

Blair, R.J.R. (1995) 'A cognitive developmental approach to morality: Investigating the psychopath.' *Cognition* 57:1-29.

Colman, A.M. and Wilson, J.C. (1997) 'Antisocial personality disorder: An evolutionary game theory analysis' *Legal and Criminological Psychology*, 2, 23-34.

De Zulueta, F. (1993*) From Pain to Violence: The Traumatic Roots of Destructiveness*. London: Whurr.

Dolan, B. and Coid, J. (1993) *Psychopathic and Anti-Social Personality Disorders:Treatment and Research Issues*. London: Gaskell.

Fischer, J.M. and Ravizza, M. (1998) *Responsibility and Control: A Theory of Moral Responsibility*. Cambridge: CUP.

Gostin, L. (1975) *A Human Condition*. London: MIND.

Hare R.D. (1980), 'A research scale for the assessment of psychopathy in criminal populations'. *Personality and Individual Differences*,1:111-117.

Hoffman, M.L. (1987). 'The contribution of empathy to justice and moral judgement', in Eisenberg, N. and Strayer, J. (eds) *Empathy and it's development*. (pp.47-80). Cambridge: Cambridge University Press.

Kohlberg, L. (1964), 'Development of moral character and moral ideology'. In Hoffman, M. and Hoffman L.W. (Eds), *Review of Child Development Research*. Russell Sage: Foundation.

Maher, B.A. (1990) 'The Irrelevance of Rationality to Adaptive Behaviour' in Spitzer, M. and Maher, B.A. (eds.)(1990), Philosophy and Psychopathology.New York: Springer-Verlag.

Mealey, L. (1995) 'The sociobiology of sociopathy: An integrated evolutionary model', collected in Baron-Cohen, S. (1997) *The Maladapted Mind -Classic Readings in Evolutionary Pschopathology*; Hove : Psychology Press.

2 Through a Glass Darkly

Ethical Dilemmas in the Treatment and Management of Psychopathic Disorder

GWEN ADSHEAD

Introduction

This chapter reviews some of the most pressing ethical dilemmas in the treatment and management of those individuals categorised "psychopathic disorder". In particular, I focus on three areas: diagnosis, treatability and preventive detention. First, in relation to diagnosis, I will look at how the philosophical and clinical literature has addressed the question, "What's wrong with psychopaths?". Second, in relation to treatability, I will suggest that "treatability" involves a number of component parts; all of which have to be considered in the analysis of this unwieldy concept. Third, in relation to preventive detention, I will argue that psychiatrists have only limited duties to third parties, and question whether these apply to the case of psychopathic disorder.

Background: why philosophy can help with psychopaths

Individuals with psychopathic disorder present particular problems diagnostically and therapeutically; they also can have a profound effect upon the staff with whom they work. Most if not all forensic clinicians appreciate that psychopathic disorder has a moral significance that other disorders do not have, and thus can generate unique ethical dilemmas. The Reed committee, when reviewing services for mentally disordered offenders, commissioned an individual report from a moral philosopher, on the nature and moral implications of the concept of psychopathy (Doyal, 1994).

Because of the moral significance of psychopathy (which I will explore in more detail below), using a theoretical approach based on moral philosophy can be practically helpful for clinicians. First, philosophy is (or can be) about analysis of concepts, like psychopathy, and whether they make intellectual sense. Second, philosophy can be about asking the right questions. Third, ethical reasoning is about coming to conclusions which are intellectually rigorous and coherent. An ethically justifiable decision is one which is based on the best quality information (drawing on empirical research), and on rigorous reasoning. Finally, a philosophical approach may help us to see when we are talking rot; a vital asset in complicated areas like psychopathy.

Definitions

One of the most common sources of confusion about psychopaths is the question of what is meant by the term itself. It is crucial to distinguish the following:

(i) Psychopathic Disorder (PD)
(ii) personality disorder
(iii) psychopath.

(i) "Psychopathic disorder"

This is a legal term, and is defined in the Mental Health Act (1983) as: "a condition resulting in abnormally aggressive or seriously irresponsible behaviour".

Psychopathic disorder (PD) is distinguished in the Mental Health Act from "mental illness", and patients are only rarely detained under both categories. This distinction is based on the long held medical view that personality disorder and mental illness are separate entities; so that in the DSM IV (American Psychiatric Association, 1994), personality disorders and mental illnesses are coded on different axes. The relationship between "Psychopathic disorder" as a legal term, and any clinical symptomatology is uncertain; in practice, it approximates to one or two kinds of personality disorder (see below).

(ii) Personality disorder

Personality disorder is a medical term, and refers to individuals with ingrained maladaptive patterns of behaviour, who also show interpersonal dysfunction of varying severity. Not all personality disordered patients could be detained under the legal category of Psychopathic Disorder; but nearly all those who are so detained have a personality disorder diagnosis. Only a few types of personality disorder are commonly associated with aggression or hostility to others; these are:

antisocial personality disorder (ASP)
borderline personality disorder (BPD)
narcissistic personality disorder (NPD).

Although other types of personality disorder may give rise to interpersonal difficulties, I assume that it is those personality disorder types which are associated with violence to others which are both clinically and morally problematic, and it is only these which will constitute "personality disorder" in this paper. Although probably most of Cleckley's "psychopaths" (Cleckley, 1941) were suffering from personality disorder, very few of them would have fulfilled criteria for the three categories identified.

(iii) Psychopath

The term "psychopath" has a life of its own, quite separate from either its legal or medical siblings. It has acquired an iconic significance; a representation of evil, in which the psychopath is one who is emotionally cold, cruel and callous. He (and in the general language it usually is he) is clever and cunning; caring nothing for the interests of others. He is usually seen as not being mentally ill in the sense of suffering, although it may often be said of him that "he must be mad". The word psychopath is frequently used in the public domain in the tabloid press, or in cinematic depictions of evil such as Dr Hannibal Lecter (in "The silence of the Lambs"). The term "psychopath" presumably derives from the concept of "psychopathy": etymologically meaningless, but now indicating a state of mind held by psychopaths. The extent to which such people actually exist is unclear.

There is enormous confusion between these three terms; particularly because those individuals who are detained under the category of Psychopathic disorder are often referred to as "psychopaths". The word "psychopathic" is also used to describe personality traits, which overlap with the concept of psychopathy, and also type of antisocial behaviour. Psychopathy is frequently used as a unitary term when clinically there are many types of "psychopath". Finally confusion is added because of the medical uncertainty about whether people **are** personality disorder or **have** personality disorders.

Diagnosis: what's "wrong" with psychopaths? (i)

There is an established literature on the nature of psychopathy, both from philosophers and well as clinicians. Some philosophers have appeared quite certain that there is something "wrong" with psychopaths (Murphy, 1972; Pritchard, 1974; Duff, 1977), and conclude that they resemble other persons with mental illnesses. It would therefore be meaningful to excuse psychopaths from full responsibility (both moral and legal) on the grounds of illness (Fields, 1996). Other philosophers have argues against both the argument about illness in the psychopath, and his/her responsibility (Haksar, 1965; Holmes, 1991; Doyal, 1994). It is noteworthy that most of these discussions take place in the context of a discussion about legal responsibility; thus placing psychopathy firmly in the realm of the criminal justice system, supporting the view that those "psychopaths" who do not act criminally do not arouse the same concern as those who do.

In contrast, much of the clinical literature has revolved around whether psychopathy and/or personality disorder are illnesses and therefore the province of psychiatry at all. Most of the clinical debates centre around the persistence of rationality in the personality disordered person; i.e there does not seem to be any defect in their capacity to reason, and that therefore they are excluded from the category of those who are mentally ill. Since personality disordered patients show neither evidence of a disease process, or suffer symptoms of an illness, they can be rejected from the clinical psychiatric realm (Lewis & Appleby, 1988).

Later authors have suggested that such patients do in fact "suffer" distressing feelings associated with their lack of successful interpersonal functioning (Norton, 1996), and may in fact have difficulties in thinking about emotions (Blair et al, 1995). Cleckley (1941) described his group os psychopaths as suffering (sic) from a type of "agnosia"; as if they did not see the effect they had on others. Derksen (1995) argues that it is better to understand personality disorder and psychopathy as difficulties and disorders of interpersonal functioning, which may then be the focus of therapeutic endeavours.

One of the principal difficulties lies in the moral significance of the "symptoms". Psychopaths are classically said to lack "empathy" for others (Cleckley, 1941; Hare, 1991). However, it is not clear whether this is a symptom or a vice. The repeated confusion of the subjective experience of being psychopathic with socially deviant behaviour adds to the uncertainty (Blackburn,1988); the very fact that it is possible to talk about psychopathy both clinically and ethically demonstrates the problem. Both early and later writers have highlighted the ethical nature of the psychopath's problems (Pritchard, 1837; cited in Blackburn 1988; Mullen, 1991).

Another source of confusion lies in the fact that there is more than one type of psychopath, and different writers see different groups of psychopaths. Those who work in forensic settings will see a different group from those who work in general out-patient settings. In a prison setting, one may find more individuals like the tabloid vision of a psychopath; in a forensic settings there may be much more overlap with metal illness, and the suffering of those with personality disorder may be more evident. In an out-patient setting, the groups may be different again; so that philosophers who draw on clinical descriptions may not have sense of the range of difficulties posed by the psychopath.

If morality is crucially about relationships; about how we think about each other, and treat one another; then it makes sense to think of psychopathy as being a deficit in relating. Insofar as it also affects action, then there may be way to understand psychopathy as type of illness, characterised by action failure (Fulford, 1989). Taking a Kantian perspective, we might understand some psychopaths as treating others "merely as a means". In psychological terms, we might think of this as an injunction not to treat others as objects; which is how many psychopaths treat their victims. It might be argued that this is the essence of lack of empathy.

What's wrong with psychopaths ? (ii)
Empathy

Harpur, Hare & Hakstian (1989) identify two factors in the make up of the psychopath:
Factor 1: Lack of empathy, callousness, narcissism.
Factor 2: Criminality, anti-social behaviour, other forms of deviance.

Although criminality and social deviance clearly overlaps with moral deviance (insofar as disobeying the law is a type of moral deviance); nevertheless, the crucial pathology of the psychopath is in the Factor 1 construct, and especially, the question of empathy.

Of the many definitions of empathy, I prefer the notion of affective resonance with the other. It contains something about the capacity to stand in another's affective shoes, which in turn entails being able to think about other people as subjects, like yourself. It is clear that empathy is involves both affective and cognitive function; what the empathy researchers have called a "hot" cognition (Miller et al, 1996). Both functions are involved, so the regulation of arousal, affect and thinking are crucial to the acquisition and maintenance of empathy.

A capacity for empathy is acquired during childhood, and is affected by early childhood experience. Of the many theories of developmental psychopathology, Bowlby's attachment theory is of particular interest in relations to psychopathy, because of its emphasis on interpersonal relating. Primates utilise attachment relationships between individuals as means to regulate anxiety in the face of threat, and that failure to make attachments in infancy can lead to attacks on own offspring, failure in social and sexual relationships, self-mutilating behaviour, and futile aggression towards others.

If violence to others demonstrates a lack of at least a type of empathy, then attachment theory suggests that failure to make attachments may contribute to failure to develop empathy. There is some limited empirical evidence to support this. Child abuse is obviously an example of failure to provide adequate care and containment for the child, and can lead to failures in attachment. For example, abused and neglected children show less interest in the distress of their play mates (Main & George, 1985).

There is some evidence that psychopaths have been exposed to adverse parenting and abuse (McCord, J. 1983; Coid 1992; Weiler & Widom 1996), and it may be that attachment failure, and a related lack of the ability to think about others, is the connection between early experience and later violence. However, it is unlikely to be a complete explanation, and there are some methodological difficulties with the research. First, there are sampling bias problems, because not all psychopaths are the same. Second, there are those who appear to be able to survive adverse parenting without becoming psychopathic themselves. Third, it may be that there are degrees of psychopathy; or psychopathy is a capacity which is more or less developed in all of us but only used to excess in a small group of individuals, who are perceived as highly deviant (remembering Cleckley's group). Perhaps psychopaths are only those who use their capacity to its fullest extent more of the time.

Lastly, it may be that, although it is possible to survive adverse parenting, there are thresholds of adversity beyond which the quality of survival is likely to be poor i.e. if physical abuse is combined with abandonment, and failure of schooling, and head injury, and poor peer skills, and unemployment and substance abuse.; then no matter how resilient the child, then full blown psychopathy is possible. Even then it may not manifest itself, except in the context of other triggers; such as a new relationship, its loss, or a stressor such as a mental illness.

Despite the incompleteness of the evidence, it does not implausible to argue that a proportion of those we call psychopaths are those who have experiences failure of parenting, of care and control; and who have developed an attachment style where avoidance of feeling is the crucial factor. This provides a framework for research, looking at empathy and parenting experiences in psychopathy.

One further difficulty remains. It seems that empathy, once acquired, can be lost, or trained out of people. A good example of this is the dismantling of empathy in those who were trained to carry out Nazi atrocities. Individuals like Franz Stangl, Commandant at Treblinka (Sereny, 1987), or those who worked in the death camps (Dicks, 1972) were trained to lose their empathy for others: by systematic desensitisation, use of affective connections to friends as self-esteem regulators, reducing personal agency and initiative. However, this profound lack of empathy towards their victims at work did not prevent them from being loving fathers, or loyal friends at home.

If a capacity for empathy is needed in order not to treat others merely as a means, then this capacity must be necessary for ethical action. However, what is to be made of a person who can exercise empathy in some situations, and not in others? He clearly has capacity; but it is not clear whether he cannot exercise it, or whether he is choosing not to. This issue of volition and autonomy has been a persistent question in relation to intention and action for philosophers and criminal lawyers; for example, in the case of Byrne [1960], we find Lord Parker,C.J stating: "the step between 'he did not..' and 'he could not...' is...incapable of scientific proof " (at p.404).

Thus empathy appears to be necessary but not sufficient for ethical action; and it is likely that there is more to find out about how psychopaths come to act unethically.

Treatability

The question of treatability arises in relation to the Mental Health Act because personality disordered patients can only be detained if they are treatable. This question relates to the previous discussion about whether psychopathy is an illness; and equally to the idea that civil liberties should not be restricted using mental health legislation unless an individual is going to be receiving help for a mental health problem.

The treatability clause raises the dilemma of which psychopath is treatable and which is not. The dilemma is made more difficult because the concept is used clumsily, and without complexity. Another difficulty arises from a rigid concept of treatability, which is not often used in general medical practice. (It may be of interest that the author's spell checker did not recognise the word "untreatable".) It may be helpful just to consider the concept in the general medical setting; for example, in relation to breast cancer. In such cases, treatability is a function of:

I. The disease: it's site, histology, it's spread.

II. The patient: her genes, her resilience, her psychological health, her social environment and family.

III. Resources: hospital waiting lists, appropriate scanners, skilled specialists and staff, professional attitudes.

IV. Science: research into aetiology and therapy.

If treatability was a function of a number of factors operating simultaneously, then it should be possible to give a much more flexible and complete account of the susceptibility of any given state or person to be treated. Note that the above model moves away from a binary treatable/not treatable; also it is affected by time, so that the combination of functions may result in a different outcome at Time 1 than at Time 2.

Treatability and psychopathic disorder: the capacity for change

Can this model be applied to psychopathy, or personality disorder? If the concept of treatability included the capacity for change, then one might see the treatability of psychopaths as a function of a number of different factors:

I. Severity of disorder: extent of dysfunction, especially affective and cognitive.

II. Personal strengths and weaknesses: therapeutic gains, family support, intelligence, early experience.

III. Hospital resources: therapists, staff support,supervision and education in the treatment of PD.

IV. Relevant research findings.

Capacity for change might be understood as high, medium or low; it also might be understood as changing over time.

If treatability is a function of many factors working together, and not just a function of the individual, then it should be possible to move the debate about treatability on to a more complex level; rather in the way that discussions about an individual's "dangerousness" have been replaced by more operational risk assessments. Using an operational set for assessing treatability means that detention could be made more ethically justifiable; for example, a personality disordered man could hardly be argued to be treatable if there were not the resources to treat him; and therefore indefinite detention in a setting without such resources would be unjustifiable.

Psychiatry and treatability

There are a number of difficulties when applying this model to psychiatric treatment, and especially to the treatment of personality disorder and psychopathy. First, the objectives of psychiatric treatment are not clear. As with other medical domains, there may be an uncertainty whether the object is care or cure. Care is traditionally not seen as part of medicine, and is the poor relation of health care services (Adshead & Dickenson). But there are more difficulties in psychiatry; such as whether the object of treatment is to make people behave better; or behave more like others? Who decides if therapy has been effective? is desirable? is necessary? The doctor? The patient? Third Parties?

When personality disordered patients are violent to others, this question of what is "wrong" with them becomes even more acute. Anxieties about public safety raise a particularly crucial question for psychiatry about its role in the control of deviant behaviour. Contrary to the Szaszian arguments about psychiatry as a covert agent of social control which medicalises deviance, violence by the mentally abnormal suggests that psychiatry has an overt role in controlling bad behaviour. Hence the recent outrage on the part of the press that dangerous paedophiles could not be detained under the Mental Health Act indefinitely for the protection of the public; and the spate of enquiries following homicides by the mentally ill.

However, if forensic psychiatrists are responsible for stopping patients behaving badly, and making them behave better, this has profound implications for the question of treatment in forensic settings. In cases of personality disorder, the patient is detained under the category of psychopathic disorder i.e. on the basis of bad behaviour. The bad behaviour does not recur because the patient is in hospital; but it is sometimes not clear what the cause of the bad behaviour is, and whether is can be "treated" (Dell & Robertson, 1992). It is also not clear, if the bad behaviour ceases, whether the patient may still have extensive psychological difficulties. The forensic psychiatrist may be asked to choose between making the subjective distress of the patient his therapeutic priority, or making risk reduction, the priority; and if risk reduction always trumps any other interest, then how can the patient's interests be protected? especially when the wider public's interests are inimical to him?

A related question is the nature and scope of the professional therapeutic duties of forensic psychiatrists. Given that they work with offender patients, are their duties different? The main question here relates to scope: do their duties extend to third parties and to what degree? And how does this relate to assessing treatability, for the purposes of detention?

Treatability dilemmas in relation to psychopathy will continue, because of the issue of public risk. The case of Mr. K. is apposite. Mr. K. is detained in a Special Hospital under the category of PD, under the Mental Health Act; despite numerous psychiatrists stating that he is untreatable. The Court of Appeal stated that the Home Secretary need not take medical advice when recalling someone, like Mr. K. to hospital. This perhaps reminds us that at present, the Mental Health Act is a useful way to preventively detain dangerous people, and the public safety issue is paramount, politically. This results in fellow psychiatrists perjuring themselves, detaining people under the Mental health Act when it is not appropriate; and a fellow citizen (Mr K.) not being treated well; perhaps merely as a means. The problem is that Mr K. is (based on his history at least) a very dangerous man; thus the dilemma remains: how far can we go in restricting the liberty of one man to keep others safe? Justification for such restriction has to be based on good quality information and judgement; and that assessment of risk and the capacity to change is a better notion than "treatability".

PREVENTIVE DETENTION: the duty of psychiatrists to third parties

As citizens we all have an interest in public safety, as well as an interest in the respect given to fellow citizens, no matter how unpleasant. Harms and wrongs done to any of us affect the community as a whole. Thus we have a commitment to appreciating both the victim and the offender; recognising the rage in the victim, and the traumatic survival of the offender.

Having a general interest, however, is not the same as having a specific professional duty. Within medicine, only public health departments have duties to communities as a whole. Even there, there is no duty to prevent disease; except insofar as this is related to a Department of Health Policy, as in current Health of the Nation targets. Even then, there is no specific duty related to individual patients; it is hoped that the rate of suicide in Nottingham will be reduced by implementing Health of the Nation Strategies, but there is no duty to reduce the rate of suicide or depression, and individuals who do become depressed will not be able to sue the health authority on the grounds that they had a duty to prevent this.

So what about harms, like aggression to others? Ethically, the prevention of harm is clearly something to be aimed for by all; but it is not some sort of ethical trump card, that can be used to justify any level of wrong. Coherent ethical reasoning demands that the justification for preventive detention of patients in hospital, solely to prevent harm to others, needs to be very strong. Otherwise, one is arguing that people like Mr. K. don't matter, and one runs the risk of treating him merely as a means i.e. treating him with the same contempt as he treated his victims. We have seen the difficulties inherent in the issue of treatability; and Mr. K is a good example, because he has said that he is not ill, and does not wish/need to have any treatment. We have thought about the problems of forcing therapy on people who do not want it; and we are aware that the courts seem to be wishing to keep a loophole open in Mental health law (by broadening the concept of treatability) so that people can be indefinitely detained; and the justification will be that of treatment.

Policemen do not have a duty to prevent harm (the recent case of Osman, not withstanding; Adshead & Morris, 1997). However, psychiatrists are currently being asked to prevent harm occurring; often by impugning the civil liberties of others. Current political weather requires psychiatrist to have duties to protect the public, in a way which conflict with their duty to serve the interests of patients. Of course, concerned professionals will have an interest, as stated above in the interests of third parties; but it is psychiatrists' professional role to tend to the ill. It is the professional role of the Home Secretary, and his departments, to protect the interests of the community; which includes those of offender patients! Previous Home Secretaries seemed to abandon the interests of offender patients altogether; and instead, opted for some vision where patients are not citizens with interests, but bodies, to be managed by professionals. Merely as a means....

It makes little sense to argue that psychiatrists have duties to prevent harm to third parties of whom they have no knowledge. Professional duties arise out of specific connections between doctors and patients; they start and close with that interaction. Psychiatrists do however have specific duties to patients, and these may be breached by considering others' interests. Psychiatrists have no political mandate to protect the public; such powers are given specifically to certain bodies like the police, because they may involve the infringement of civil liberties. Practically, psychiatrists are not trained in the detection and prevention of crime; they are also not contracted to do so, nor indemnified to do so.

It makes even less sense in relation to the management of personality disorder, and psychopathy. The strongest argument for psychiatrists preventing their patients from doing harm is in the case of psychotic patients, who are arguably not competent to make decisions. In such cases, it might be justifiable to make another person (eg a psychiatrist) responsible for their actions. The case is even stronger when they are detained i.e. it makes sense to apportion responsibility if the patient escapes, and harms someone. But in relation to PD, where basic competence is preserved, it seems hard to justify. One might argue that they are not morally competent (pace Mullen, 1991); but then one might counter-argue that this simply begs the question of whether anyone can be morally competent for another. How could such an argument be sustained; especially if moral agency is what makes us persons at all? Such an argument would suggest that individuals can not be persons, and others, as it were, "hold" their personhood for them.

Conclusion

There are a considerable number of difficult dilemmas in the management of psychopathy. It seems to me that moral philosophy and clinical reasoning can join forces to try and take the analytic process forward; to achieve better and better answers, that reflect the complexity of situations and connections between people. Empirical research and better conceptual handling are crucial for coming to good quality ethical decisions. Nevertheless, the issue of public safety, and the anxiety it causes, is likely to continue to confound the process, and this may mean that moral philosophy and clinical psychiatry will also have to be engaged politically.

References

Adshead, G. & Dickenson,D. (1993) 'Why do doctors and nurses disagree?', In Dickenson, D. & Johnson, M. (eds,) *Death, dying and bereavement.* Open University: Sage.

Adshead, G. & Morris, F. (1997) The liability of psychiatrists for the violent actions of their patients. *New Law Journal.* American Psychiatric Association (1994) *Diagnostic and Statistical Manual* Version IV. Washington: American Psychiatric Press.

Blackburn, R. (1988) 'On moral judgements and personality disorders: the myth of psychopathic personality revisited'. *British Journal of Psychiatry*, 153: 505-512.

Blair, J., Sellars, C., Strickland, I, Clark, F., Williams, A, Smith, M. & Jones, L. (1995) 'Emotion attributions in the psychopath'. *Personality and Individual Differences*, 19: 413-437.

Cleckley, H.(1941) *The Mask of Sanity.* St. Louis,C.V. Mosby. 5th edition 1988.

Coid, J. (1992), 'DSM-III diagnosis in criminal psychopaths: the way forward.' *Criminal Behaviour and Mental Health*, 2: 778-79.

Dell. S. & Robertson, G. (1988) *Sentenced to hospital: Offenders in Broadmoor.* Maudsley Mongraph 32: Oxford: Oxford University Press.

Derksen, J. (1995) *Personality disorders: clinical and social perspectives.* Chichester: John Wiley.

Dicks, H.V. (1972) *Licensed mass murder: a socio-psychological study of some SS killers.* Sussex University Press; Chatto: Heinemann.

Doyal, L. (1994) 'Notes on the moral problems of diagnosing and treating psychopathic personality disorder'. In Report of the Department of Health and Home Office *Working Group on Psychopathic Disorder.* London: Department of Health. Annex B.

Duff, A. (1977) Psychopathy and moral understanding. *American Philosophical Quarterly*, 14: 189-200.

Fields, L. (1996) Psychopathy, other-regarding moral beliefs and responsibility. *Philosophy, psychiatry and psychology*, 3: 261-278.

Fulford,K.W.M (1989) *Moral theory and medical practice*. Cambridge: Cambridge University Press.
Haksar, V. (1965) 'The responsibilty of psychopaths'. *The Philosophical Quarterly*, 15: 135-145.
Hare, R. (1991) *The Hare Psychopathy Checklist Revised.* Toronto Ontario: Multi health Systems.
Harpur, T., Hare, R & Hkastian, A. (1989) 'Two factor conceptualisation of psychopathy: construct validity and assessment implications' *Psychological Assessment,* 1: 6-17.
Holmes, C. (1991) 'Psychopathic disorder: a category mistake?' *Journal of Medical Ethics*, 17: 77-86.
Lewis, G. & Appleby, L. (1988) 'Persoanlity disorder: the patients psychiatrists Dislike'. *British Journal of Psychiatry*, 153: 44-49.
Miller, P., Eisenberg, N., Fabes, R. & Shell, R. (1996) 'Relations of moral reasoning and vicarious emotion to young chhildren's prosocial behaviour towards peers and adults'. *Developmental Psychology*, 32: 210-219.
Main, M. & George, C. (1985) 'Responses of abused and disadvantaged toddlers to distress in age-mates: a study in a day care setting'. *Developmental Psychology*, 21: 407-412.
McCord, J. (1983) 'A forty year perspective on effects of child abuse and Neglect'. *Child Abuse and Neglect*, 7: 265-270.
Mullen, P. (1991) 'Psychopathy as a disorder of ethical action'. *Criminal Behaviour and Mental Health.*
Murphy, J. (1972) 'Moral death: a Kantian essay on psychopathy'. *Ethics,* 82: 284-298.
Norton, K. (1996) 'Management of difficult personality disorder patients.' *Advances in psychiatric treatment*, 2: 202-210.
Pritchard, M. (1974) 'Responsibility, understanding and psychopathology.' *Monist*, 58: 630-645.
Sereny, G. (1974) *Into that Darkness*. London: Andre Deutsch.
Weiler, B.L. & Widom, C. (1996) 'Psychopathy and violent behaviour in abused and neglected adults'. *Criminal Behaviour and Mental Health*, 6: 263-281.
Legal Cases. Byrne [1960] 2QB 396-405.

3 Freedom, Resentment and the Psychopath

PIERS BENN

The condition referred to by the modern term 'psychopathy' has exercised philosophical and legal brains ever since the invention of the term 'moral insanity' by J. C. Prichard (Prichard, 1835), which describes a condition that is commonly identified with it. Of course, in popular usage 'psychopathy' refers to something imprecise, and popular images, reinforced by tabloid newspapers and television dramas, of madmen and violent maniacs tend to mislead. In the popular imagination, psychopaths are deranged and fearsome. They are responsible for many of the more horrific and well-publicised murders and assaults, and are thought to be a breed apart from the class of 'normal' criminals, in that they are peculiarly vicious and dangerous. Prichard's term 'moral insanity' accords with this public perception: the things they do are thought to be so brutal and wicked that the agents cannot be considered genuinely sane.

A pressing psychiatric issue turns on the proper classification of the condition, and the question of what sense, if any, it can be seen as a disorder. Does the term 'psychopathy' refer to a natural kind, a class of beings with some common nature? Or is the term - as many reasonably suspect with respect to some psychiatric classifications - a reference to a merely nominal kind, devised to suit our particular needs and interests? This is a reasonable question when it comes to such concepts as psychosis and delusion. For example, what it is that makes a certain unusual and fiercely held conviction a delusion, rather than an 'ordinarily' irrational or ill-founded belief, is a moot issue. It is plausible that the concepts in question are cluster concepts or Wittgensteinian 'family resemblance' notions, with at best fuzzy boundaries and no defining set of necessary and sufficient conditions for their application. But these concepts do not only raise problems of psychiatric classification. With respect to psychopathy, some of the most interesting and intractable questions are moral ones. One of the most intriguing concerns the moral dimensions of 'moral insanity'. The idea of insanity suggests a disorder, or a rational incapacity, that might be susceptible to treatment, but the qualification 'moral' hints at something we would naturally contrast with psychiatric disorder: namely, a freely chosen condition for which the agent is morally responsible, and properly susceptible to praise and blame. As an hyperbolic description of extreme wickedness - analogous perhaps to 'insane' foolishness - the idea of moral insanity is, perhaps, intelligible. But construed more literally as behaviour which reveals a rational incapacity, it becomes doubtful that it can be described in moral terms at all.

Participant Reactive Attitudes

My chief concern is with certain moral questions raised by the psychopathic condition. Specifically I am interested in psychopaths' moral responsibility for their actions and lives, and the kind of moral claims upon the rest of us that they might have. But I begin with a fruitful way of looking at the whole question of responsibility, and our moral reactions to moral agents. My starting point is the well-known contribution of P.F. Strawson to the problem of freedom and responsibility, made in his acclaimed lecture 'Freedom and Resentment' (Strawson, 1962). This classic contribution was in part a response to discussions current at the time about the implications of determinism for our normal ascriptions of responsibility to ourselves and others, and the moral and personal concepts at the heart of meaningful interpersonal lives. In contrast with other dominant positions in the dispute about free will and determinism, Strawson suggests that our commitment to certain 'participant reactive attitudes' neither is nor should be the outcome of any theoretical position. Rather than clearly identify his position with that of libertarians, compatibilists or hard determinists, Strawson reminds us first of all of our pervasive commitments to the participant attitudes in question, and the reasons we invoke whenever we modify or abandon them in particular cases.

The point of reminding us of the centrality of these participant attitudes in our shared social world is partly to focus our minds on what we would be giving up if we accepted a thesis, such as determinism, and became theoretically convinced that the truth of this thesis entailed that these attitudes were irrational.

Such participant attitudes include not only the 'moral' ones such as disapproval, guilt or admiration, but a whole range of responses that depend on our valuing, as well as evaluating, persons. Strawson mentions self-esteem, vanity and forgiveness, in addition to moral reactions such as resentment. We could add to this list such things as love, sexual desire, friendship, respect, jealousy and contempt. Reactions of this sort, whether or not we approve of all of them, are a seemingly essential component of the realm of intentional understanding in which we lead meaningful lives. Strawson admits that the 'decay' or 'repudiation' of such attitudes would not be self-contradictory. But he adds at once: "...I am strongly inclined to think that it is, for us as we are, practically inconceivable. The human commitment to participation in ordinary inter-personal relationships is, I think, too thoroughgoing and deeply rooted for us to take seriously the thought that a general theoretical conviction might so change our world that, in it, there were no longer any such things as inter-personal relationships as we normally understand them;..." (Strawson, 1962 p.68 in Watson, 1982). And this observation is consistent with another observation, concerning the grounds we have for abandoning specific reactive attitudes in particular circumstances. If we decide to withhold resentment towards someone whose behaviour would in normal circumstances justify resentment, it is because we have detected some local, particular abnormality about the case in question. Perhaps we have discovered some excusing or mitigating factor, such as the fact that the person in question is under unusual stress. Perhaps, in other cases, we have discovered some abnormality in the agent and not just in his temporary circumstances: if we conclude that he is psychotic, or extremely immature, or brain-damaged, we cease to experience the usual participant attitudes that we would normally form towards those who behave in similar ways. We adopt instead an 'objective' attitude to him, regarding him as a possible object of study or analysis rather than an agent with who we can genuinely engage. We may have to fight him if he threatens us, but we cannot quarrel with him. Special factors such as these only highlight the indispensability of the framework itself. The normality of the attitudes is taken as given, and we need special reasons if we are to set them aside.

Strawson notoriously goes on to suggest that questions about the 'rationality' of the participant attitudes as such, as opposed to particular attitudes on particular occasions, can occur "only to one who had utterly failed to grasp the purport of our natural human commitment to ordinary interpersonal attitudes. This commitment is part of the general framework of human life, not something that can come up for review as particular cases can come up for review..." (Strawson, 1962, p. 70 in Watson, 1982). Now this, quite understandably, has led some readers to think that Strawson has treated the whole issue somewhat evasively. It is all very well pointing out, with considerable justification, that the framework of participant attitudes is both practically indispensable and, in a certain sense, an essential ingredient in valuable social and moral relations. It is quite another to claim that this settles the problem of their rationality. Think of philosophical scepticism - a comparison used by Strawson in defence of his case. It is one thing to say that no one can take radical scepticism seriously, at least outside of a philosophy seminar. It is quite another to suggest that, for this reason, scepticism ought not to be taken seriously. Perhaps we are doomed to irrationality, in both cases?

This disturbing possibility cannot be ruled out - even if the knowledge that it cannot be ruled out has no effect on our individual judgements. But our commitments to reactive attitudes are so deeply rooted that we ought, at least, to be suspicious of any argument whose conclusion is that we should stop viewing ourselves in this way. One reason for this is Kantian. The 'idea' of freedom is seemingly forced upon me, at least from a first-personal perspective. Questions of what I ought to do are forced upon me as a condition of being an agent at all; I cannot fail to see myself as faced with practical questions. And whatever reactive attitudes I form about myself, such as pride or guilt, are an inseparable part of my own sense of agency. Reactive attitudes directed towards others are similarly based on the belief that they too face practical questions in the way I do. And this begins to explain why it is that certain sorts of people are generally exempt from the framework of participant responses. Small children, for example, and the genuinely psychotic, can at most partially be members of that framework. For they can participate only partially, if at all, in our shared moral and social world. Reason, including practical reason, presupposes the possibility of dialogue, whether with others or in the form of 'internal debate'. But meaningful dialogue with, for example, the severely deluded is beset with grave obstacles. For such people do not fully share our world. All normal people, obviously enough, have different values, beliefs and life-experiences, but there is a deeper sense in which we must share our world if real communication is possible.

'Normal' wrongdoers

This, at last, brings us to the main subject of this paper. Given that we can agree that certain types of individual are excluded from the full range of participant attitudes, precisely because they cannot properly participate in a shared moral world, what should we say of psychopaths? Is there a moral or social world that we can share with them? If psychopathy is nothing but another term for extreme moral delinquency, then we might think we do share such a world. For serious moral flaws do not seem, in themselves, to rule out mutually comprehensible moral dialogue, as the following examples suggest.

First of all, take the sufferer from weakness of will or *akrasia*. Such a person seems an obvious case of someone who understands moral dialogue well enough, since he reproaches himself for falling short of standards that he accepts in principle. The condition does, it should be admitted, raise some very familiar puzzles, but I do not think akratic people need exhibit insincerity in the moral judgements they make. Those who take an externalist view about the relationship between assent to moral norms, and intention-formation, will probably deny that there is even a *prima facie* mystery about akrasia; or they might say that if there is insincerity, it is not about the assent to a moral principle or standard, but rather the commitment to acting according to it. But it is possible to be perfectly sincere in your assent to 'let me do X', even if, in conflict states, that commitment is overridden by a desire to do something else. Incidentally, we should not assume that there is only one explanation for akrasia: explanatory parsimony does not always yield true answers, and there may be a variety of explanations applicable on different occasions. But there are some cases of akrasia where moral awareness is perfectly well in place, and when it is both possible and right to engage in fruitful moral dialogue with the akrates.

Next, it appears that even those who do bad things for moral reasons they misguidedly take to be good, can participate in such dialogue and grasp some central moral concerns. Such people may misunderstand the real nature of a certain virtue or vice, and act wrongly as a result, but a certain nominal understanding may still be present. People who take the advice that 'one must be cruel to be kind' so much to heart that their cruelty overshadows the kindness intended, can still have some understanding of kindness, even if it is misapplied. Furthermore, their nominal understanding of kindness can have motivational power. As we shall see, in this they differ from psychopaths, whose nominal understanding of moral concepts extends little further than their ability to feign moral concerns, and has no motivational pull at all.

A third example would be someone whose life, in many respects, is lived well, and according to moral concepts sufficiently grasped, but who has some major flaw, perhaps so reinforced by habit that his moral grasp of the fault in question is weak or non-existent. Perhaps he is honest and fair in his dealings with strangers but neglects his family, taking their presence and support for granted. In this case, we might conclude that moral dialogue about showing love to those closest to him, is almost impossible. Still, we might rightly hold him responsible for this flaw, since he has no general lack of moral understanding, and he could acquire understanding of his obligations to his family if only he considered how this could be derived from what he already knows. There is also a fourth type of morally flawed person, whose difference to the psychopath is more germane. Imagine someone who pursues relentless and obsessive projects of revenge, out of a distorted moral conviction. Perhaps she feels aggrieved about a humiliation she endured, or a violation of her rights; perhaps she is driven by strong envy of another person, whose success she persuades herself is undeserved, and desires to see this person brought down. Now she may be shrewd and calculating in her plans, as some 'primary psychopaths' as described by Cleckley (Cleckley, 1976) are said to be, but she is driven by motives that are alien to psychopaths in significant ways. For wounded pride, resentment, envy, and *schadenfreude* all seem to be Strawsonian participant attitudes, even if not very admirable ones. And they often require some understanding of moral concepts, if only because they sometimes need to masquerade - to the self as well as to others - as morally grounded.

This thought should now be combined with another: that (or so it seems to me) only beings capable of participant reactive attitudes can be proper objects of such attitudes. We do not resent dangerous dogs when they cause mayhem, but we do resent burglars when they steal or harm our property. We lament the effects of natural disasters, but we feel indignant at the harm deliberately caused by some anti-social people. And one reason for this reaction is that we take malicious or other objectionable people to have intolerable attitudes to their victims. Not only do they harm them, but their actions express, or spring from, attitudes like contempt; they seem to regard their victims as unworthy or of little account. Our indignation towards such people is very often provoked in circumstances where the harm they do is trivial. We get angry with queue-jumpers because we detect in them an attitude of contempt for others: an attitude expressible as 'I matter more than you'. The attitude, rather than the deed as such, is the object of the resentment.

The psychopath as non-participant

Now there is strong evidence that psychopathy is a condition distinct from that of the common-or-garden criminal or ordinarily anti-social person. For example, it is likely that at least some psychopaths are not driven by hostile reactive attitudes.[1] Rather, they are frequently deficient in many or even all reactive attitudes, and lacking in both empathy and antipathy. The point about empathy is interestingly made by Elliott and Gillett in their analysis of the moral defects of psychopaths: "They are defective in their empathy with others because interpersonal factors do not properly enter into their intentional activity, and they do not recognise the impact and implications of their actions for others. Psychopaths cannot form fully informed 'reactive attitudes' based on the attitudes, needs and vulnerabilities of others" (Elliott and Gillett, 1992, pp 65-66). And a related point is made by Duff: "...we cannot find in a psychopath's life any intelligible dimension of value, emotion or rational concern: and this lack is logically connected to an inability to understand this dimension of the lives of others; there is a close logical connection between two commonly identified features of psychopathy: firstly, that it involves an incapacity for such emotional and moral responses as love, remorse and concern for others... Secondly [a psychopath], although not intellectually incompetent, is unable properly to understand the "nature and quality" of his acts, since he cannot grasp those emotional and moral aspects which are as much a part of them as their empirical features." (Duff, 1977 pp. 191-92).

Lack of empathy on this scale naturally provokes indignation and resentment from those at its receiving end. But psychopaths' disengagement from others, and their failure to display the sort of hostility that springs from inappropriate and egoistic *self-evaluation* (as opposed to simple, unreflective egocentricity), should make us reconsider the moral responses that come naturally to us. For it is equally important that psychopaths are frequently indifferent to the consequences *for themselves* of their anti-social behaviour. Paradoxically, although in a certain way they are abnormally self-centred, yet they are also highly impulsive and disinclined to pursue long-term goals. Indeed, it may well be that they have no long-term goals. Considerations of prudence do not weigh with them as they do for 'normal' anti-social people, and many criminal psychopaths are caught simply because of their lack of care in covering their tracks. Now it is plausible that there is a connection between this lack of prudence, and deficiencies in self-evaluating attitudes, such as self-esteem, pride and self-love. For one important factor underlying prudence, at least when it extends significantly beyond simple fight-or-flight mechanisms, is a set of concepts to do with self-worth. There is more to normal prudence than a simple desire to feel happy in the future; prudence concerns itself more with the shape of your life as a whole and the coherence of its narrative, than with ensuring that, during any given future segment of your life, you will experience feelings of satisfaction and that these feelings will be serially reproduced over time. We might therefore expect people seriously lacking in prudence to lack the sort of self-concern, including the *amour-propre* or personal pride, that motivates normal people both to pursue their long-term interests and, on occasion, to entertain hostile attitudes towards others.

We should of course be careful not to overstate this point, since the unpleasant attitudes that make us indignant when we are at the receiving end of them (like the contempt shown by the arrogant) do not wholly depend, for their existence, on these concepts of self-worth. But I think there is still a significant connection between them. The impulsive, disjointed and imprudent aspects of psychopathy, which are explained by psychopaths' lack of genuinely self-evaluative concepts, diminish their capacity to experience the full range of participant reactive attitudes. If this is correct, and if it is also correct to suggest that only creatures able to form these attitudes are proper objects of such attitudes, then we have a good reason for holding that psychopaths are, at least to a significant extent, outside the range of appropriate objects of these Strawsonian reactions.

Why, though, is it that only creatures able to form participant attitudes are proper objects of such attitudes on the part of others? We reach an answer if we consider the usual ways in which these attitudes are expressed, and what the point of expressing them is. Take, as a central example, anger. Anger is a participant response, one of whose purposes is to induce fear in its recipient, and it is inspired by a perception of such things as injustice or cruelty. Of course, we often say we feel anger at misfortunes that we rationally acknowledge to be no one's fault, but in such cases we tend to personify the causes of the misfortunes. Even when the appropriate emotion is frustration or annoyance rather than anger, we often cope better if we imagine there has been an intentional wrong, and become imaginatively involved in fighting this wrong, in much the way that we imaginatively become engaged with certain emotions when watching a play. Whatever the psychological or evolutionary *explanations* of anger, it is *intelligible* chiefly as a disposition to attack and try to defeat an agent of injustice, or of a comparable wrong. That is, it is more than a disposition to undo the effects of the wrongful deed: in Hegelian terminology it is a disposition to annul the *wrong* (Knox, 1976). But there can be wrongs only where there are wrongdoers, and annulling a wrong must involve confronting the perpetrator, usually in an indignant fashion, with his responsibility for it. It is for this reason that those retributive acts that are the natural expression of moral anger and serve to propitiate it, succeed only if they are understood *as* retributive. So retribution, and in general acts that express anger, are essentially communicative. They confront the wrongdoer as a rational and free agent with what he has done, and try to get him to understand its true nature. This helps us see why anger is a *participant* response: it makes sense only as something communicated between participants in a basically shared moral world.

The aim of expressing such responses is to induce in another such reactions as fear, guilt or remorse. Such expression may take the form of punishment, although more often it is purely verbal. But as a communicative act, it has a point only if its message can be understood. If psychopaths really are denied, as Duff puts it, the requisite moral understanding, and lack certain emotional and evaluative dimensions to their lives, then to that extent psychopaths are not proper objects of these responses. To at least some degree, they cannot be considered real participants. And if, as some experiments seem to indicate, psychopaths are largely immune from fear or anxiety, then when we express our anger to them we achieve little more than the cathartic satisfaction of venting spleen. As far as inducing fear or similar reactions goes, we might as well get angry with menacing rottweilers, or - like the hapless Basil Fawlty - scream at and beat our cars when they fail to start.

Earlier on we stressed that the only proper targets of the Strawsonian attitudes are individuals able to form at least some of them themselves. Perhaps we should clarify this by adding that the potential to form these attitudes during a normal course of development, as well as the present ability to form them, can be enough to justify an individual's inclusion in the Strawsonian web. In any case, it is the either the ability, or the potential, to form them, rather than actually having formed them, that is important here. For example, children have both a limited participant understanding and the potential for greater understanding. Their acquisition of the greater understanding obviously takes time. But it is by being treated as though they already had greater moral understanding than they actually have, that they come to increase that understanding. It may be right to be indignant with a child for something she has just done, even if she did not have much understanding of the nature of what she did; she may not have known it was wrong, but she comes to know it by experiencing adults' reactions.

Psychopaths (some of whom, for all we know, may be children!) present different problems. For psychopathy seems to be an *incapacity* and not just a lack in one's life of certain emotional and moral dimensions. In some ways it seems analogous to autism.[2]

Autistic people have great difficulty understanding certain social meanings, such as are contained in facial expressions or in nuance, and although they may be able to learn social rules that help them get along, it is doubtful that they ever really internalise or fully grasp their underlying rationale. Psychopaths similarly, or at least the 'primary' ones (the glib charmers), possess a certain superficial grasp of morality: they know that certain kinds of behaviour are socially unacceptable, and their plausibility depends on their ability to assume certain moral demeanours such as remorse. But they are unable to understand certain moral (and perhaps prudential) concepts at an appropriately deep level, or to absorb such understanding and be automatically guided by it. In fact I suspect there are interesting parallels to be explored between psychopathy and the more profound sorts of hypocrisy, and the manner in which psychopaths understand moral concepts bears some similarity to that of deeply hypocritical people (see Benn, 1993).

Psychopathy and the 'rational amoralist'

We have seen that authors like Duff suggest that psychopathy is a disorder, manifested in an inability to understand a central dimension of normal life. This incapacity is not a matter of the psychopath being unable to live a moral life, or understand moral concepts, even if he tried; it is rather a matter of him having no conception of what would count as trying. Its source is not lack of strength but lack of understanding. This leads to another interesting contrast. Imagine a 'rational amoralist' philosopher who, after carefully examining various arguments concerning the metaethical status of moral obligations, has concluded *both* that there are no objective values,[3] *and* that it is inconsistent with this thesis to maintain any moral convictions. Maybe there are a few such philosophers, but it is (let us hope) far-fetched to consider them psychopathic. It is implausible that intellectual arguments like these could deprive us of the affective dimension of human life that is at the core of moral motivation and conviction - or in short, deprive us of the understanding that the psychopath already lacks (unless such arguments are a psychopathic rationalisation of a pre-existing condition!) A sincere philosophical champion of radical moral scepticism - that is, normative as well as metaethical scepticism - would probably end up in a position similar to philosophical sceptics about induction or the external world, who consider themselves unable to give up the very convictions that they announce to be philosophically indefensible. A Strawsonian resort to the fundamental 'given-ness' of both epistemological and moral conviction, and the absurdity of thinking they could or should 'rationally' be abandoned, would probably be the most inviting option in such cases. By contrast, it seems unlikely that the psychopath has any theory of morality that leads him to embrace a doctrine of nihilism.

Incapacities and their causes

But now we should say more about the incapacity itself, as there is much opportunity for confusion about how such incapacity removes (or partially removes[4]) psychopaths from the network of participant reactive attitudes. The thrust of my argument so far has been, as is evident, inspired by Strawson, and I have tried to suggest that psychopaths, admitted by most writers not to be insane or lacking in intelligence, should still to some extent be regarded as Strawson says we should regard the insane and the exceptionally immature. With most mental illness, the central concept is that of incapacity: conditions like schizophrenia and manic-depression can be seen as incapacitating their sufferers, at least to some extent, from normal functioning. What the mentally ill are incapable of doing is a moot point, which goes to the very heart of our concept of illness. A plausible neo-Aristotelian suggestion is that illness of any kind impedes the flourishing of the body or mind by preventing it from operating in accordance with its distinctive function. To specify what activities or functions constitute such flourishing would be to invite needless controversy, and for this reason we should be content with a schematic rather than detailed account of illness and incapacity. In the case of psychopaths, the incapacity is one of understanding, and it entails a lack of engagement in any real moral dialogue with others, and a failure to participate in a shared moral world. Since blame and punishment are fundamentally communicative, they fail in their aims when it comes to psychopaths.

Now this point should be contrasted with the commonly expressed view that it is the *cause* of the incapacity that matters, when it comes to deciding whether to regard psychopaths as morally blameworthy for their deeds. Some authors make much of the brain abnormalities that certain psychopaths are said to display. Some relevant research is laid out by Elliott and Gillett (Elliott and Gillett, 1992), who cite evidence of abnormality of frontal lobe activity in psychopaths, which indicates impaired attention and response to environmental conditions which are relevant to forming complex intentions. The authors tell us that "psychopaths have different cerebral processes in complex conditions which require that one inhibit certain responses, apply oneself to a task and modify one's behaviour according to a considered judgement about a situation." Moreover, "both primary and secondary psychopaths' brains show a relative inability to process information about future response requirements where these involve responding or refraining from responding in order to avoid punishment" (Elliott and Gillett, 1992, p. 63). Other research includes that of the American psychiatrist Dorothy Lewis, who has spent twenty years examining violent criminals, and Jonathan Pincus, a neurologist at Georgetown University, Washington.[5] Their joint research convinces them that there is a systematic connection between criminal violence and various neurological disturbances, including frontal lobe dysfunction and an abnormal stress response system. They also link criminal behaviour with childhood abuse and neglect, which they say can cause entire cortical structures never properly to develop. The cocktail of brain abnormality and abuse during childhood is often lethal, and a strong indicator of violent criminality in adult life.

Now the linkage of brain abnormalities with anti-social behaviour is an empirical matter of considerable interest. But some theorists draw questionable conclusions from it. Lewis, for example, holds that these violent criminals are not evil, but damaged; they are not, or not fully, morally responsible for their actions precisely because their brain abnormalities make it impossible for them to think and behave as normal members of society. And this view echoes a common and attractive view that even if violent behaviour always has causes, there is something decisively exculpating about *physical causes in the brain*.

Now there are two problems this view raises. The first is simply about causation. That certain brain abnormalities can be closely correlated with a psychopathic or anti-social personality does not in itself show that there is a causal connection. Why not say that the brain abnormalities are the physical aspect of a psycho-physical condition?

Moreover, if some type of physicalism is true, as most philosophers of mind believe, then all mental events are physical, and at least on one level of description may be subject to bio-chemical laws. The correlation of brain abnormalities (or better, non-typical features?) with deviant personality does not show that the individuals in question are not responsible for their actions, any more than physical/mental correlations show the same for any normal person. But what Lewis and others are driving at, I think, is that there is something *incapacitating* about certain brain abnormalities: if your frontal lobes are dysfunctional, then that stops you from developing a normal personality, just as having very short legs stops you from running very fast. And this point has much credibility. But it brings us to the second problem with the exculpatory account. For the physical cause or base for the condition is not itself the decisive exculpating factor; it is not the fact that the incapacitating cause is a physical condition of the brain that matters. Rather, what matters is the psychological condition itself, specifically, that the psychopathic state renders impossible the kind of moral communication that takes the form of praise, blame, rewards and punishments.

A disturbing possible implication

Still, this view will produce some tensions. The participant attitudes, as Strawson says, are a condition of meaningful personal life and neither could, nor should, be dislodged by theory. And it is this stress on the unavoidable 'given-ness' of these attitudes that might also incline us, in spite of the arguments I have outlined, to include psychopaths in the realm of participant attitudes. For there is still the appealing thought that 'psychopathy' and its cognates are pseudo-clinical terms that disguise a fundamentally moral condition. It is hard, surely, not to feel resentful and angry when victimised by such people. The very fact that they are sane and intelligent reinforces the conviction that they are part of our moral world, even though they have coldly and knowingly rejected its precepts (see Bavidge and Cole, 1995). In addition, bearing in mind the plausible thought that psychopathy is not an all-or-nothing condition, but has degrees, there may for that reason be room for qualified moral reactions towards them.

However, I wish briefly to open up, for final reflection, another way of recognising the force of this point. This is to follow Jeffrie G. Murphy (Murphy, 1972) in suggesting that if certain people really do lack fundamental moral capacities, they thereby lose their entitlement to be treated as having a full set of rights. Starting from the Kantian thought that only autonomous moral beings are 'ends in themselves', we might come to regard psychopaths as so far from fulfilling this requirement, that our treatment of them is no longer governed by normal Kantian requirements of respect for persons. For Kant and his followers, persons, as embodiments of the moral law, demand our absolute respect and may not be treated as mere means, whereas to try to treat non-persons - for example, animals, which are sentient but which lack the crucial moral capacities - as ends in themselves would mark a fundamental mistake about their nature. In fact, the very attempt would reveal the mistake at once: there can be no such thing as gaining a cat's consent for 'euthanasia', for example. This idea is echoed in Kantian formulations of contractualist theories of morality. The guiding thought here is that morality is that set of principles that rational agents could freely agree to observe, on condition that everyone else observe them as well. And commitment to such an agreement entails a commitment to reciprocity. If certain individuals are incapable of understanding the need for reciprocity, or of entertaining the moral feelings that normally motivate its observance, then for that reason they exclude themselves from the agreement, and may be treated in ways in which normal people may never treat one another.

In spite of its liberal credentials, in the classical sense of the word, this seems in some ways to be a harsh, illiberal thought. However, it seems to follow from a combination of a Kant-inspired theory of moral obligation, and an apparently 'liberal' recognition that psychopaths might not be blameworthy because they are incapable of certain moral concerns. If they are genuinely incapable, then what is the basis for extending such concern to them? Of course, we should not forget crucial moral considerations that are not distinctively Kantian: concerns of sympathy and virtue, for example, which forbid the infliction of needless suffering (whatever counts as 'needless'), and prohibit certain uses of the individuals in question, just as virtue plausibly forbids certain uses of animals. Moreover, were we to try to enact a policy of excluding psychopaths from the realm of rights, we would have to think extremely hard about problems of psychiatric classification, of 'slippery slopes' and of the effect on society's sensibilities of such a policy. But I think the general idea focuses upon the surprising implications of a seemingly liberal policy. If we reject these implications, but accept the reasoning from the premises, then we shall have reason to re-consider the view that psychopaths are not bad, but damaged. We might then find ourselves back with the moralistic view of psychopaths, which thinks of psychopathy as a misleading synonym for moral wickedness.

However, even if there is a liberal temptation to misclassify certain people as psychopathic, who are in fact perfectly capable of the moral understanding necessary for responsibility, I have tried to suggest that there probably is a condition of moral incapacity which is distinct from ordinary delinquency. And though I have no answer to the question of how people with this condition should be dealt with, we are led back with renewed urgency to the perennial enquiry as to the proper basis for the everyday assignment of rights and responsibilities.

Notes

1 My basic thesis is that the psychopathic condition often involves a significant lack of certain reactive attitudes, and that this has interesting moral implications for our treatment of psychopaths. But I did not want to overstate the case, since there are probably people with marked psychopathic traits who do entertain at least some of these attitudes. We should remember that psychopathy, like moral responsibility, probably admits of degrees. We should also bear in mind that even if a marked absence of at least some of these attitudes is a frequent hallmark of psychopathy, it need not be a necessary or sufficient condition for it.

2 Carl Elliot pointed out this analogy to me in correspondence.

3 I am stating this thesis loosely: more specifically, it could be the claim that all versions of moral realism and moral objectivism are false.

4 Though I have not often seen this point made, it strikes me as plausible that psychopathy is a matter of degree, although most of the cases discussed concern people quite near the extreme end of the spectrum.

5 See the science report on 'The Criminal Brain' in The Independent Magazine, 4 May 1997 p.19ff.

References

Bavidge, M and Cole, M. J. (1995) 'Is Psychopathy a Moral Concept?', in Almond, B. (Ed), *Introducing Applied Ethics*. Oxford: Blackwell. pp.185-196.

Benn, P. (1993). 'What is Wrong with Hypocrisy?' *International Journal of Moral and Social Studies,* 8, No. 3. pp.191-2.

Cleckley, H. (1976). *The Mask of Sanity.* St. Louis: MI.

Duff, A. (1977). Psychopathy and Moral Understanding. *American Philosophical Quarterly,* 14, No. 3.

Elliott, C. and Gillett, G. (1992). 'Moral insanity and practical reason.' *Philosophical Psychology* 5, No. 1. pp. 65-66.

Knox, T. M., ed. (1976). *Hegel's Philosophy of Right.* Oxford: Oxford University Press.

Murphy, J.G. (1972). ' Moral Death: a Kantian Essay on Psychopathy.' *Ethics* pp. 284-98.

Prichard, J. C. (1835). *A Treatise on Insanity.* London: Sherwood, Gilbert and Piper.

Strawson, P. F. (1962), Freedom and Resentment. *Proceedings of the British Academy* xlviii: 1-25. Reprinted in Watson, G., (ed.) 1982. *Free Will,* Oxford: Oxford University Press. pp. 59-80.

4 Disordered Minds, Diseased Brains and Real People

K.W.M. (BILL) FULFORD

"Madness is a subject that ought to interest philosophers; but they have had surprisingly little to say about it" Anthony Quinton, 1985

In the dozen or so years since Anthony Quinton wrote these words we have seen an unprecedented explosion of cross-disciplinary work between philosophy and psychiatry. There are now frequent national and international meetings; some 25 academic groups have sprung up in different parts of the world (the Philosophy Group in the Royal College of Psychiatrists has over 1200 members); and the subject has a well established international journal, *Philosophy, Psychiatry and Psychology**. Both psychiatric and philosophical organisations have supported these developments: in the UK, The Royal College of Psychiatrists, The Society for Applied Philosophy, and The Royal Institute of Philosophy, have all been active in this respect. Support has come also from the universities, with MA and PhD programmes now running at Sheffield, Warwick, and, most recently, King's College in London. The latest endorsement has come from the *Philosopher's Index*, the premier citation index for philosophy, which has recently added "philosophy of psychiatry" to its list of recognised philosophical sub-disciplines.

---

*Published by the Johns Hopkins University Press for the British and American groups for philosophy and psychiatry.

There are no doubt many and complex reasons why the philosophy of psychiatry should have taken off at just this time. A key reason, though, taking Quinton's prescient point, is straightforwardly that philosophers and psychiatrists have a lot to learn from each other. One embedded topic of this book, responsibility, is very much a case in point. For philosophers, responsibility is an aspect of what in the popular imagination at least is the mother of all philosophical problems, the mind-body problem - how to reconcile free agency, traditionally an aspect of mind, with the deterministic machinery of brains. For psychiatrists, a key aspect of this problem is the undermining of responsibility by mental disorder. This covers issues of "mad or bad?" in forensic psychiatry and the corresponding "mad or sad?" issues raised by involuntary psychiatric treatment. None of this is hot news, of course. What *is* new, though, and giving a new edge of urgency to cross-disciplinary work in this area, is developments in the neurosciences. Advances in neuropharmacology and genetics are filling out our understanding of the biological basis of mind. Dynamic brain imaging is allowing us for the first time to look directly into the workings of the brain, to see the brain in action. Such developments are raising anew, and in a peculiarly acute way, the traditional "problem of responsibility".

In this chapter I want to consider some of the issues raised by cross-disciplinary work between philosophy and psychiatry on responsibility. Many of the chapters of this book are concerned with psychopathy. This is a category of mental disorder in which issues of responsibility, of "mad or bad?", are writ large: people suffering from psychopathic personality disorder are, so it is said, indifferent to social and moral norms; but are they thereby bad (voluntarily breaching these norms) or mad (unable to recognise and/or act on them)? In this chapter, however, I will be considering a very different kind of case, one of brain tumour. Such cases have traditionally been taken to be paradigmatic of legally excusing conditions (the behaviour of the person concerned is perceived as being "driven by" their brain tumour). What we will find, though, is that even in such cases the mind cannot be written out of the clinical picture. This is essentially because above in such cases, it is not just a brain with which we are concerned, nor even just a mind, but a real person.

I will start with a note on the methodology of cross-disciplinary work between philosophy and psychiatry. This will then lead straight into our case history, that of a real person (I am calling her "Mrs Lazy") written up in The Times newspaper. I will consider Mrs Lazy's case in three stages, a mind-only stage, a brain-only stage, and a mind-plus-brain stage. As we will see, the first two stages correspond broadly with the positions of traditional anti-psychiatry and of traditional psychiatry. It is from the third stage, the mind-plus-brain stage, that the significance of Mrs Lazy's status as a real person will emerge. In a brief concluding section I will indicate the wider significance of Mrs Lazy's case for responsibility and for cross-disciplinary work generally in philosophy of psychiatry.

A Note on Method

First, then, methods. Philosophy is a notoriously multi-faceted discipline and there are correspondingly many ways of skinning the philosophy of psychiatry cat. One fruitful approach is top down, i.e. drawing on philosophical theory to illuminate practical problems in psychiatry. In my own work I have drawn on aspects of moral theory - work by R M Hare, G J Warnock and others on the logical properties (the meanings and implications) of value terms (Fulford, 1989, chs 2-5). Although not originally concerned with psychiatry, moral theory in the hands of such philosophers has a whole series of implications for clinical work and research in psychiatry (e.g. Fulford, Smirnoff and Snow, 1993; Jackson and Fulford, 1997).

A second approach is bottom up, i.e. starting not from theory but from practice. This is how the argument will run in this chapter. Instead of looking to philosophical work on the mind-body problem to help with the practical problems raised by responsibility, brain scans, and so on, we will start with the practical problems and see where they lead for the mind-body problem. This is of course broadly in the J L Austin tradition of linguistic analysis, or ordinary language philosophy, a tradition which, although still perhaps unfashionable in philosophy is making something of a comeback (e.g. Hallen and Sodipo, 1997). The basic idea is straightforward enough: we are often better at using concepts than defining them (try defining 'time' if you doubt this), so why not study our use of concepts as a guide to their meanings?

I have argued elsewhere that linguistic analysis is *prima facie* relevant to psychiatry in a number of respects (Fulford, 1990). In the present case its importance is that it gives us a broader or more complete picture of the key concepts of disorder used in psychiatry. As a former Professor of Psychiatry at the Maudsley Hospital, the late Sir Denis Hill, pointed out (personal communication), linguistic analysis is in this respect like psychoanalysis: both are consciousness-raising exercises. Austin used this feature of linguistic analysis to help identify a series of distinctions built into the broad notion of an 'excuse', this in turn being a way of investigating responsibility as an aspect of agency (Austin 1956-57).

In psychiatry, linguistic analysis can help us to become conscious of aspects of our conceptual scheme which we have (partly) suppressed because of their (perceived) inconsistency with the demands of natural science: insight (Fulford, 1989, ch 10), evaluative delusions (Fulford, 1991), psychosis (Fulford, 1994), and the evaluative element of meaning in our concepts of disorder generally (Fulford, 1989, Chapter 3), are all cases in point. In this chapter, similarly, linguistic analysis will help us to become aware of aspects of the concept of mind (particularly as related to responsibility) which, although not recognised for what they are, are nonetheless crucial to the way we understand and respond to what appears to be a "brain only" case. As we will see, this has important consequences, theoretical and practical.

Linguistic analysis, as Austin himself was at pains to emphasise, is not an end in itself. It is no more than one way of getting started with some kinds of philosophical problem (see generally a number of quotes in Warnock, 1989, especially pp.s 4-6). The constraints generated by careful linguistic analysis of clinical case reports may help to structure and drive theory forward. But just which kinds of philosophical theory are pertinent in a given case can only be finally determined *post hoc*. An exciting and challenging feature of the philosophy of psychiatry is that just below the conceptual problems with which it is concerned are many of the deepest problems of general metaphysics (freewill, for instance, is just below the surface of the clinical problem of attributing responsibility). In psychiatry, moreover, Continental and Anglo-American philosophies, for so long separated, are in principle equally important and in practice often complementary. I will not be pursuing any of the rich connections opened up between philosophy and psychiatry by linguistic analysis in this chapter. It is important to be aware of them, though, and I will return to them briefly in my conclusions. So, let's "get started" with the case of Mrs Lazy.

The Case of Mrs Lazy - Part I - Antipsychiatry has its (Mind-Only) Say

On Monday September 2nd 1996, The Times newspaper carried a report by its medical correspondent, Jeremy Laurance, in the Home News section, under the headline *Lazy Wife has her Head Examined.* We will be looking at Jeremy Laurence's report in three parts. The first part ran as follows:

> *A houseproud woman who decided she was fed up cleaning and preferred to watch television had to defend herself to doctors who feared that she was ill.*
>
> *The 55-year-old housewife argued that her change of habit was entirely reasonable after decades of looking after the family home. Doctors in the neurology department of the Radcliffe Infirmary, Oxford, agreed with her husband that her personality change required investigation...*

Although Mrs Lazy is presented anonymously, she is a real person. Later on in Jeremy Laurence's report he indicates that her case was written up originally in the British Medical Journal. So this is not a philosopher's invention. Indeed it was not thought of as a 'philosophical' case at all. It was a problem in medical diagnosis. Mrs Lazy, as the report describes, had undergone a change in personality which led her husband and the doctors to believe that she was ill and "required investigation".

Yet if we read this first extract with an eye sharpened by J L Austin's emphasis on the importance of ordinary language, it is a rich source of observations about the use of mind-body concepts in relation to questions of health, illness and disease. Indeed with just these first two paragraphs we go right to the heart of the mind-body problem. Mrs Lazy is introduced as a free agent who 'decided' she was fed up with housework. Anti-psychiatry, therefore, would identify closely with the phrase that follows - she "had to defend herself" to doctors who, with what could reasonably be regarded as an unwarranted extension of the concept of illness, "feared that she was ill". Thomas Szasz was among those who led the way in claiming that mental illnesses are not brain diseases but, straightforwardly, "problems of living" [Szasz, 1960]. This is an extreme claim for a condition like schizophrenia, perhaps. But psychiatric diagnoses are notoriously vulnerable to abusive use as a means of social control (in the former USSR, for example, see Fulford, Smirnoff and Snow, 1993); and Szasz's work has been aimed precisely at reasserting our responsibility for our 'problems of living' as free agents.

In Mrs Lazy's case, moreover, the anti-psychiatry charge against her doctors seems strengthened by the fact that her 'defence' does indeed look reasonable - many women, after decades of housework, decide it is time to put their feet up, or to branch out in some other direction. Reasonableness, as a mark of responsibility, has recently been endorsed by our own courts (in the UK) in the case of C [Re C, 1994]. C was an elderly man, an ex-sportsman, who refused amputation of his gangrenous leg because he delusionally believed that he was a surgeon whose opinion was more reliable than those of his doctors. The courts upheld his right to refuse on the grounds (inter alia) that, however irrational his reasons, such a decision would not be unusual in someone of his age and background. (In fact, he recovered!) Imagine, then, the reaction had Mrs Lazy decided to "defend herself" against her doctors in court, citing the case of C.

We get a quite different picture, though, if we put on our clinical spectacles and think of Mrs Lazy, not as someone with a 'problem of living' but as someone who might be ill. Instead of an existential re-alignment, instead of a down-trodden housewife throwing off the shackles of domesticity, we see a woman with a change in personality suggesting the diagnosis of "frontal lobe syndrome". In this condition the personality of the person concerned shows a characteristic shift towards fecklessness and irresponsibility.

Mrs Lazy's behaviour could be viewed in this way. It would then be a symptom of damage to the frontal lobes of her brain (i.e. the front part of the brain just behind the forehead).

Moreover, Mrs Lazy's husband's concerns are highly relevant in this respect. From an anti-psychiatry perspective, he is viewed as being motivated by the need to control his wife: her decision is medicalised and therefore invalidated, making her subject to interventions designed to control her deviance, to bring her back into line. But parents, as any family doctor will tell you, are often very good at knowing when their children are really ill, even if, at the time, there are no obvious or well-defined symptoms. Why not a husband, therefore?

So, how do we square the circle? One practical course is to get Mrs Lazy's agreement to a brain scan. This is a non-invasive procedure and one which is likely to show if there is anything wrong (such as a tumour) about which something can be done: tumours in this part of the brain are often "silent" clinically, i.e. they show no signs or symptoms (apart sometimes from loss of the sense of smell in one nostril, due to pressure on the nerve tracts in the brain running from that side of the nose). In fact, a brain scan was done. The second extract from the case of Mrs Lazy records describes what was found.

Mrs Lazy - Part II - Biological Psychiatry Has its (Brain-Only) Say

Mrs Lazy's story as written up in The Times continues thus,

...They (the doctors) were right. A brain scan discovered a tumour the size of a grapefruit. The surgeon who removed it said it was the largest he had seen. Called a meningioma, it is thought to have been growing for at least 15 years.

Mike Hanna, the neurologist who examined the woman, said: "She was referred to us by her GP because of her husband's concerns. Although her views were perfectly reasonable, we had to take account of her husband's views and those of her family and friends who insisted her behaviour was out of character...

Mrs Lazy, then, did indeed have a large tumour in her frontal lobes which was successfully removed. At first glance, this outcome fully vindicated her doctor's original concerns, and indeed those of Mrs Lazy's husband, family and friends. As a *practical* aspect of the mind-body problem, therefore, Mrs Lazy's story certainly illustrates the dangers of an ideologically driven anti-psychiatry. There are important issues (about patient autonomy, etc.) to be considered before deciding to intervene surgically even granted the presence of a tumour. But to have simply neglected the *possibility* of a frontal lobe tumour on the grounds that all mental disorders are "problems of living", would have been negligent.

Mrs Lazy's story thus contradicts anti-psychiatry, at least of the extreme Szaszian kind that would make mental illness a myth. Szasz would no doubt reply that Mrs Lazy had a *brain* disease. Many psychiatrists, too, although diametrically opposed to Szasz, would take an equivalent line. This is surprising at first sight. But the current strongly "biological" orthodoxy in psychiatry would see Mrs Lazy's case as paradigmatic of the way psychiatry will develop as its scientific basis becomes more secure. Brain science, biological psychiatry assumes, *modern* brain science, will lay bare the mysteries of the mind. It will reveal the causal disease processes underlying mental disorders and thus make possible new medical treatments; not, perhaps, old fashioned leucotomies and ECT (electro-shock therapy), but (we may imagine), precisely targeted physical manipulations by designer drugs, laser scalpels, nano-technological robot probes, silicon-chip prosthetic implants, and the like. Until recently these were science fiction. But advances in the neurosciences have brought such treatments within the bounds of technical possibility in the early decades of the new millennium.

Faced with such serious conditions as schizophrenia or intractable depression, few would deny the need for new and more effective treatments. This is why patient organisations, like the National Schizophrenia Fellowship in the UK and the National Alliance for the Mentally Ill in the USA, are among those who strongly support the biological turn in psychiatry. But the very importance of these developments, promissory as they still are, has led to what John Locke would have called "enthusiasms". One such enthusiasm is a false, or at any rate hazardous, extrapolation from conditions like schizophrenia, for which only the most extreme anti-psychiatrist would deny the value of treatment, to other more equivocal cases, not least personality disorders such as psychopathy.

A second and perhaps less creditable 'enthusiasm' among biological psychiatrists, is a false separation between physical and psychological approaches to the management of mental disorders. The American psychiatrist, Edward Shorter, for example, concludes his scholarly history of psychiatry with a clarion call for a future of brain-based interventions, writing off psychotherapy as 'aimless chat' (Shorter, 1997). Mrs Lazy's story would suit his purposes. Psychotherapy, even if indicated in her case, would have been 'aimless chat' so far as her frontal lobe tumour was concerned. But the underlying assumption that we can in principle do everything that is needed in psychiatry with some variant of brain surgery is clearly flawed. It is flawed *clinically*: Mrs Lazy, we must hope, had the benefit of counselling as well as of surgery. It is also flawed *pragmatically*: as biological psychiatrists readily acknowledge there are still technological barriers to a brain-based future, and some form of 'talking therapy', combining behavioural and psychotherapeutic elements, is likely to remain the treatment of choice for some time to come for a whole range of less serious disorders. It is flawed *scientifically*: modern neuroscience fully accommodates the physiological effects of psychological and social processes. It is flawed, above all, *conceptually*: The comprehensive reduction of mind to brain, on which the hopes of biological psychiatry for 'physical treatments for all' depend, requires that talk, no less than surgery, be capable of changing brains, albeit in somewhat different ways!

The dangers of the false separation of mind and brain in biological psychiatry are well illustrated by the history of psychosomatic concepts in medicine. It is not so long ago that biologically-minded doctors were inclined to deny that a patient's state of mind could influence the state of their body. How, it was argued, could feeling sad for example, possibly alter the blood supply to the heart (increasing the risk of a heart attack), or affect the healing of a surgical wound. Nowadays this seems positively antediluvian! Not only do we have a well-established concept of psychosomatic disorder but some of the causal pathways between the psychological and the physiological are beginning to be well understood. Interestingly, one of these pathways is the pineal gland, the organ by way of which René Descartes, the seventeenth century French philosopher responsible for the mind-body problem in its present form, speculated that mind and body might interact.

Descartes: the First Biological Psychiatrist?

Descartes' identification of the pineal gland as what we might now call a mind-body transceiver is often treated as something of a philosophical joke. As a *brain*-body transceiver, though, and in this sense as a conduit between the psychological and physical, it was a reasonable hypothesis. The pineal gland is a pea-sized organ situated more or less in the centre of the head with a cord or stalk of nervous tissue connecting it directly with the deep parts of the brain. In Descartes' time it had no obvious function and to all appearances it could well have been a mind-body transceiver. This construal, it is worth noting, would require qualifying the nature of Descartes' mind-body dualism.

Descartes' arguments aimed to show the distinctness of mind and brain. But if mind and brain interacted in the way he suggested, this would make the mental turn out to be in one sense *physical,* i.e. in the sense that anything which is causally interactive within the physical realm is itself *part of that realm.* This would still be different from arguing that mental states are really states of the body. The mind, for example, perhaps like the signal arriving at a TV set, could be a distinct field interacting with the body through the brain (Colin McGinn has suggested something along these lines [McGinn, 1993]).

All the same, there is a clinically important sense in which Descartes' hypothesis about the pineal has turned out to be right. For the pineal is now known to be, if not the connection between mind and body, at least an important conduit between the *brain* and the rest of the body (there are others, e.g. the autonomic nervous system). The pineal secretes a wide variety of hormones which influence the state of the body; these secretions are under the control of higher centres in the brain which mediate emotional and other psychological functions (including the reception of signals from the outside world); these psychological functions, in turn, are influenced by the hormones stimulated (directly or indirectly, i.e. via the bodily changes they produce) by the pineal. All this falls firmly within the remit of the biological sciences.

Brain-body Dualism and Psychiatric Disease Classification

Descartes' hypothesis about the pineal, reinterpreted as mediating *brain*-body dualism, thus anticipated the development of biological psychiatry and, indeed, a range of modern biomedical disease categories such as 'psychosomatic disorder', 'endogenous depression', 'psychogenic pain' and 'organic psychosis'. Such categories are often taken to reflect mind-body dualism. This has been noticeably so in the debate between psychiatrists and anti-psychiatrists about the validity of the concept of mental illness. Thomas Szasz, for example, accused psychiatry of conflating mind and body, of an invalid assimilation of mental disorder (illness) to physical disease [Szasz, 1960]. Arguing on the other hand for psychiatry, Sir Martin Roth and Jerome Kroll accused Szasz in his turn of an old fashioned and philosophically unsound dualism [Roth and Kroll, 1986]. Yet psychosomatic disease categories need express nothing more mysterious than the idea that the *brain* interacts with the rest of the body.

We can see this by reconstructing psychosomatic categories in terms of brain-body dualism. For example, *psychosomatic disorders* become bodily diseases caused or made worse by those states of the brain which mediate psychological functions (e.g. ulcerative colitis, a severe bowel disease, is often aggravated by long-term anxiety); in this sense, then, 'psycho-somatic' disorders are no more mysterious than what we might call 'dermato-hepatic' disorders - i.e., skin disorders caused by states of the liver (e.g. jaundice). Similarly, *endogenous depression* becomes depression which arises from an internal influence on the (putative) parts of the brain mediating sadness, as against reactive depression which arises from external influences (e.g. bereavement) on these same brain parts (the distinction is not at present clinically useful because the symptoms and current treatments of depression are largely independent of the aetiological relationship to outside events).

Then again, *psychogenic pain* becomes pain (itself a brain state) caused by changes in those parts of the brain which mediate psychological functions (as distinct from its usual cause in external noxious stimuli). Finally, *organic psychoses* become psychotic disorders caused by gross pathology (tumour, endocrine disorders, reduced blood supply, etc) affecting the brain. Whereas *functional*, or *non-organic*, psychoses (e.g. schizophrenia) are caused by more subtle (and still putative) changes in the fine structure of the parts of the brain mediating psychological functions.

With brain-body dualism of this modified Cartesian kind, then, biological psychiatry could encompass a good deal more than some of its own enthusiasts recognise. An effective biological psychiatry does not depend on debunking psychological treatments. There are, no doubt, issues of professional territory here. But an effective biological psychiatry, like the neurosciences on which it draws, should accommodate rather than exclude psychological and social processes. Derek Bolton and Jonathan Hill, in their recent *Mind, Meaning and Mental Disorder* (1996), have worked out a detailed theory, drawing broadly on a representational theory of mind, of how this might be done.

Is brain-body dualism, then, expanded in scope in this way, sufficient for the purposes of psychiatry? Mrs Lazy's case, from what we have heard thus far, might seem to suggest that it is. But let's look at how her story turned out.

Mrs Lazy - Part III - Mind and Body

The concluding part of the case of Mrs Lazy was written up in The Times as follows,

...Dr Hanna, who sent a copy of the scan to the British Medical Journal, said: "Nine times out of ten, someone who undergoes a personality change will have a depressive illness. One time in ten, or less, something may be going on in their brain." The benign tumour at the front of her brain was pushing aside the frontal

lobes. The tip of the lobes are known to be where aspects of personality such as drive and motivation reside.

Two months after surgery, she has not recovered her enthusiasm for house-work. Dr Hanna said: "If the tumour had gone on growing, she would almost certainly have died. The pressure may have changed her personality for good.

The outcome of the story, then, was that despite the removal of her tumour, Mrs Lazy did not regain her enthusiasm for housework. What are we to make of this? Clinically, the causal story offered by the doctor, Dr Hanna, is entirely plausible. It is *possible* that the tumour was merely incidental to Mrs Lazy's change of personality and the anti-psychiatry lobby might want to press this point. As noted earlier, though, tumours in this part of the brain (the frontal lobes) are known to produce changes in personality of just the kind shown by Mrs Lazy (the frontal lobe syndrome); and it is not unreasonable to believe that after 15 years this large tumour (the largest the surgeon had ever seen) could indeed have affected Mrs Lazy's frontal lobes "for good".

At one level, therefore, this remains an obvious 'brain case'. The brain subserves personality. A change in personality is thus to be understood as a change in the brain. There is a clear (linguistic-analytic) signal, though, even in this brief report, that the mind side of the mind-body problem cannot be so easily eliminated. This signal comes in the penultimate paragraph of the article, in Dr Hanna's reference to depressive illness. A change in personality, he is reported as saying, is usually due to a "depressive illness", but in perhaps less than one case in ten "something may be going on *in their (the patient's) brain*" (emphasis added). Depressive illness, then, *versus* brain disease? But biological psychiatry, as we have seen, rightly emphasises the brain basis of depressive illness. If pressed, Dr Hanna would no doubt want to say that he was speaking loosely and that "of course" mental illness has a brain basis. But what he is reported as actually *saying* implies a contrast between mental illness and brain disease.

This is highly significant from the point of view of linguistic analysis. As noted earlier (in the *Note on Method*, above), linguistic analysis, careful observation of ordinary usage, aims to make us more aware of the concepts structuring the way we organise and understand the world around us. Dr Hanna's comment, then, rather like a Freudian slip, reveals hidden meanings. It reveals aspects of the mind carried by the concept of mental disorder which, even in a 'brain case' like Mrs Lazy's, are not carried by the concept of brain disease.

We could read Dr Hanna's comment negatively, as revealing a prejudice against the mental summed up in such phrases as "all in the mind". Mind, according to this prejudice, and with it mental illness, is somehow 'unreal', whereas the body and bodily diseases are 'real'. The rejection in principle of 'talking therapies' by some biological psychiatrists is no doubt driven in part by this prejudice. There is also a positive reading of Dr Hanna's comment, though, according to which mental illness, in addition to all the "psychosomatic" possibilities carried by brain-body dualism, brings within the scope of medicine those properties of mind which, as Colin McGinn (1982, p16) has put it "invite us to distinguish the mental realm from the physical" - phenomenal consciousness, a "point of view", and, not least, freedom and responsibility.

Philosophically, it remains an open question whether some form of non-reductive monism can accommodate the 'mental' properties of mind. Mrs Lazy's story, however, as we will now see, shows that in psychiatry at least, the distinctively mental aspects of the mind remain important even in those cases that appear to be most obviously brain-based. In the remainder of this paper I want to consider some of these 'mental' aspects in particular through the importance of patients' experiences of illness.

Patients' Experiences of Illness

Clinically, one effect of medicine's focus on the body has been a relative neglect of patients' experiences of illness. This is bad medicine. Whatever the power of modern diagnostic techniques (like brain scans), good clinical care still depends on careful attention to each patient's experience as a unique individual.

Philosophically, of course, this lands us right in the deep end of the mind-body problem: phenomenal consciousness, qualia, first and third person references, having a 'point of view', and so on are all just below the surface of this apparently straightforward clinical principle. Descriptive psychopathology, however, as the study of the symptoms of mental disorders is known in psychiatry, offers a relatively tractable area for cross-disciplinary work between philosophy and psychiatry in the study of the structure of consciousness.

Modern descriptive psychopathology is based largely on the work of the philosopher-psychiatrist Karl Jaspers in the early years of this century. There are parallels between Jaspers' period and our own. Jasper's wrote his foundational 'General Psychopathology' (1913a) in part as a reaction against what he perceived as the unrealistic ambitions of the biological psychiatry of that period. New histological techniques had led to the description of a number of brain lesions. The identification of GPI (general paralysis of the insane) with syphilis was a major advance. But then, as now, psychiatrists were too quick to generalize from this success. They had unrealistic expectations for what could be done with a brain-only approach which Jasper's sought to counter-balance by redirecting their attention back to the mind.

Psychiatry has made steady progress through this century in defining the symptoms of mental disorder using the framework of ideas set out by Jaspers. Modern structured interview schedules for eliciting and describing the "mental state", such as the PSE (Present State Examination; Wing, Cooper and Sartorius, 1974), have given us reliable methods as a basis for scientific work on mental disorders. Yet neuroscience itself is now forcing us to revisit the foundations of our psychopathology. Dynamic brain imaging has given us access to the brain in action; but this has brought with it the problem of relating what we see "in the brain" to what is going on "in the mind". The last few years have thus witnessed an explosion of what the American philosophers George Graham and Lynn Stevens have called "philosophical psychopathology" (Graham and Stephens, 1994).

Philosophical psychopathology has all the marks of a Kuhnian paradigm shift. The framework of ideas developed by Jaspers has guided psychiatry through a period of steady scientific growth and development. But we have now reached the point where a new framework is needed. Just what this framework will look like remains to be seen. But we can anticipate a little from current trends. It seems likely, for example, that it will draw equally on Continental and Anglo-American analytic philosophical sources: exemplars of the latter include Braude (1991), Clark (1996), Glover (1988), Radden (1996); and specifically on responsibility, Braude, 1996; but recent work has also returned to the philosophical roots of psychopathology in Continental phenomenology (Philpott, 1998; see Mishara et al., 1998 for a recent review).

This double-barrelled approach, combining Continental and Anglo-American analytic methods, could be good for psychiatry. Jaspers' psychopathology has been the basis for the development of an essentially explanatory science to which Anglo-American analytic philosophy is sympathetic. But Jaspers himself emphasised that psychopathology demands understanding as well as explanation, the identification of meaningful as well as causal connections (Jaspers, 1913b). As Adshead argues in this book, this is highly relevant to attributions of responsibility and other problematic aspects of the diagnosis and assessment of personality disorder (Chapter 2 above). It is also crucial in a more general way to good clinical care. Just as doctors have tended to neglect patients' experiences of illness, so they have tended to neglect the meanings of these experiences to the people concerned. Taking a blood test, for example, or doing a mental state examination, are assumed to be sufficient for "medical" purposes. But this leaves the patient as a unique human being out in the cold. In The Times article about Mrs Lazy's case, it is remarkable how quickly her perspective drops out of the story. This is a brief case report. It may well be that in practice the clinical team were engaged fully in Mrs Lazy's perspective throughout. But this is certainly not reflected in the way her story is actually told. After the opening lines, Mrs Lazy (as a person) disappears. We see her brain but we do not see her. This is just how many patients particularly with mental disorders do feel - invisible as individual people - when faced with health professionals (see, e.g., Read, 1996, and Campbell, 1996).

The double-barrelled approach could also be good for philosophy. A growing number of philosophers now recognize that the split between Anglo-American and Continental methods, although dominating philosophy for much of this century, is ill-adapted to modern philosophical concerns. Philosophical psychopathology offers an important testing ground for a combined approach. This is partly because, as just noted, psychopathology actually *requires* both kinds of philosophy. It is also because of the wide variety of kinds and conditions of mental disorder encompassed by psychopathology. This is illustrated by the conceptual map of psychiatry shown in the Figure. Austin first pointed out (at the end of his 'A plea for Excuses', 1956-57), and as Kathy Wilkes (1988) has recently argued in detail, the heterogeneity of psychopathology is a valuable resource for philosophy. So much so that Stephen Toulmin (1980) suggested psychiatry could well become the epicentre of philosophical work on mind and brain.

The Parts of the Map and the Map as a Whole

If the heterogeneity of psychopathology is a resource for philosophy, it is also a constraint on philosophical theory. Any account of responsibility, for example, must explain, or at any rate be consistent with, the very distinct ways in which, say, a person with psychopathic personality disorder, a patient with dementia, and one who is deluded, are all in different ways and to different degrees not responsible; and how indeed all of these differ from 'organic' cases such as epileptic automatism. Mrs Lazy's case illustrates the demands on theory here. She is introduced as someone firmly on the left of the map, in the area of moral problems. She ends up firmly on the right of the map, as an organic 'brain case'. Dr Hanna's slip about "depressive illness" shows that had she not turned out to have a brain tumour, she might have ended up diagnosed as suffering from a mental disorder and hence somewhere in the middle.

Philosophical psychopathology, therefore, must be concerned with the distinct parts of the conceptual map of psychiatry. It must give an account of the diversity of mental disorders. The account may be positive, helping us to unpack and come to a better understanding of the different kinds of psychopathology. This is important in its own right and also as it bears on our understanding of issues such as responsibility. Or the account may be negative, showing that the locations on the map, and hence the intuitive shifts of location in cases like Mrs Lazy's, are illusions, a 'folk psychology' equivalent.

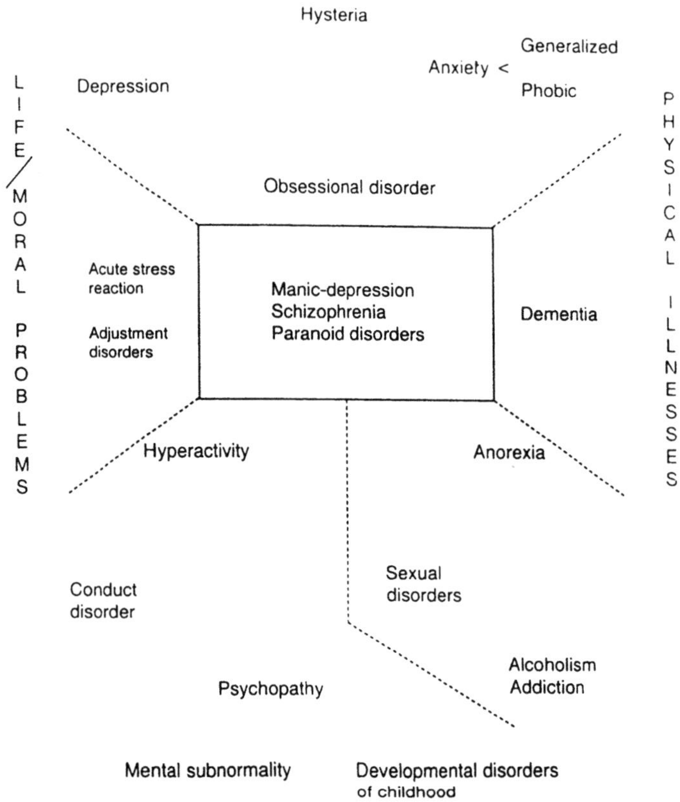

The map illustrates diagrammatically how the different kinds of psychopathology form a conceptual bridge between moral problems (broadly on the left of the map) and medical problems (broadly on the right). Thus, hysteria is conceptually close to malingering, alcoholism to drunkenness and psychopathy to criminality, whereas dementia is closer to physical disease to pre-scientific 'folk physics'. But as a constraint on theory, philosophical psychopathology must engage one way or another with the variety of mental disorders.

If the parts of the map are important in philosophical psychopathology, though, so too are the features of the map as a whole. A key feature of the map, as the Figure shows, is that our concepts of mental disorder provide a bridge between mind (the moral problems on the left of the map) and brain (the bodily disorders in the right of the map). As Mrs Lazy's case illustrates, antipsychiatry in effect collapses psychopathology as a whole to the left, while biological psychiatry (narrowly conceived) in effect collapses it to the right. Philosophical psychopathology, by contrast, must provide an account of this feature of the map as it stands. As with the parts of the map, the account may be negative or positive, but an account there must be. Current trends suggest that the account will be positive and that it will draw particularly on two areas of philosophy which in recent years have been relatively low on the philosophical agenda, agency and values. I want to look briefly at both of these.

Agency and Values in Psychopathology

Much of the work over the last twenty five years in medicine and psychiatry on concepts of disorder, taking its cue from natural science, has been concerned with disturbances in the functioning of bodily and mental parts and systems (Fulford, 1989, Chapter 1). A broadly similar bias has until recently been evident in philosophy of mind (Fulford, 1993a). Recent work, though, has suggested that there are aspects both of our general concepts of disorder (Nordenfelt, 1987) and of specific areas of psychopathology (e.g. delusion, Fulford, 1989, Chapter 10; and thought insertion, Stephens and Graham, 1994, and Chadwick, 1994), which are more readily understood in terms of disturbances of action, i.e. of the characteristic mode of activity not of bodily and mental parts and systems but of agents as a whole. And in relation at least to responsibility, as several chapters in this book indicate, the relevant "unit of analysis" is surely persons as agents, whatever insights may be derived from studies of their component parts and systems. In philosophy of mind, too, there has been a recently renewed interest in agency (see, e.g. Campbell 1994, and Luntley, 1998). There is common ground here, then, and with the developments in neuroscience noted earlier already acting as a catalyst (Bolton, 1998; also Gindro and Mordini, 1998), it seems likely that we will see some exciting developments here over the next few years.

Values, similarly, have been prominent in recent work on concepts of disorder. One reason for this is clear from the Figure. Conditions on the right of map (in bodily medicine) may appear value free, but those on the left are overtly value-laden. Personality disorder is a case in point. Even in the self-proclaimed scientific classifications of modern psychiatry, such as the ICD-10 (WHO, 1992) and the DSM-IV (American Psychiatric Association, 1994), personality disorder is not only value-laden but actually defined by reference to social-evaluative norms (Fulford, 1994).

Many of the early attacks on the concept of mental disorder were driven by this feature of the conceptual map of psychiatry. Szasz (1960) explicitly, and others implicitly, took the value-laden nature of mental disorder as an indication that it was different in kind from bodily disorder (that it was a moral not a medical problem). More recently the argument has been about whether the evaluative element in mental disorder can be written out by redefining it descriptively (see, for example, the debate between Wakefield, 1995, and Sadler and Agich, 1995). The debate about mental illness has thus become a *forme fruste* of an even longer running debate in theoretical ethics, the so-called "is-ought" debate. The latter debate, like work on agency, has been well down the philosophical agenda. But as I have shown elsewhere (Fulford, 1989), the is-ought debate is a rich source of illumination for the debate about mental illness. It shows, in particular and crucially, that while values are indeed endemic to our concepts of disorder, bodily and mental, the more value-laden nature of *mental* disorder reflects the fact that psychiatric diagnosis differs from diagnosis in bodily medicine in being concerned with areas of human experience and behaviour - wish, desire, belief, etc.- *in which our values are characteristically and legitimately diverse*.

There is not the space here to go into this in detail. The essential point, which I take most directly from R M Hare (e.g. in 1952 and 1963), is that a value term (such as "illness") may come to have largely descriptive connotations (as in the case of "bodily illness") where the descriptive criteria for the value judgement it expresses are largely agreed upon, whereas its connotations will remain largely evaluative (as in the case of "mental illness") where there is no such agreement (see Fulford, 1989, Chapters 3, 4 and 5, for the applications of this to medicine and psychiatry).

Value theory, as the more abstract part of ethics is sometimes called, is clearly relevant to our understanding of attributions of responsibility. Interestingly, though, it has been relatively neglected by the philosophy of mind. Values, so far as I am aware, rarely figure in lists of the "mental" aspects of mind produced by non-reductionist philosophers (Colin McGinn, for example, does not mention them). This is in marked contrast to philosophical action theory, which, although now firmly part of the philosophy of mind, used to be part of ethics; and it was part of ethics precisely because of its connections with agency and responsibility (for example in the work of J L Austin). Yet the *prima facie* links between "values" and "mind" are evident enough: the link between aesthetic judgements and an individual's unique point of view, for example, and indeed between moral responsibility and freedom. Perhaps, then, philosophical psychopathology, spanning as it does between mind and brain, will prove to be the conduit through which values follow agency into the philosophy of mind.

This could be a crucial development, a truly radical change of paradigm, for philosophy. It would certainly be a crucial development for psychiatry. Productive as the traditional medical model has been in psychiatry, its emphasis on scientific facts has carried with it a failure to recognize the importance of values. This has been (relatively) unimportant in physical medicine because, as noted above, the values concerned in attributions of bodily disorder, at least in "high tech" areas of acute medicine, are largely agreed upon and hence, to this extent, unproblematic in practice. Of course, there are many areas even of physical medicine in which diversity of values is important: in relation to gender and body image, for example; and in the whole range of issues of treatment choice covered by traditional 'medical ethics'. But the diversity of values involved in our psychopathological concepts means that values are practically important *throughout* psychiatry. This is not just a matter of theory, moreover. Values were important, for example, in the high profile abuses of psychiatric diagnostic concepts in the former USSR (Fulford, Smirnoff and Snow, 1993). But they are important also in the widespread dissatisfaction among many patients with psychiatric services (Campbell, 1996). And they are important, not least, neuroscientifically, in a range of key diagnostic distinctions (for example between religious experience and psychosis, Jackson and Fulford, 1997, and in cross-cultural psychiatry, Fulford, 1998).

Diversity of values is important diagnostically throughout psychiatry, then. Mrs Lazy, again, makes the point. As we saw earlier, once her brain tumour was diagnosed, her case seemed to offer a clear example of the power of a value-free, scientific medical model. This was how it was reported. The Times newspaper article, like the doctors concerned, assumed that the tumour had damaged her frontal lobes, making them *under*-active. But why should we assume this? Perhaps her frontal lobes had been *over*-active before the tumour appeared. Perhaps Mrs Lazy had been pathologically conscientious about her housework and the tumour had *cured* her. There is a revealing (though no doubt unintentional) play on words in Dr Hanna's conclusion that the "pressure may have changed her personality *for good*". He meant *permanently*. Mrs Lazy may have said "for the *better*".

Conclusions

In this chapter I have explored some of the issues about responsibility, itself an aspect of the mind-body problem, as raised by the story of a real person, Mrs Lazy, reported in The Times newspaper. This has illustrated the value of a straightforwardly Austinian linguistic analytic methodology in the new cross-disciplinary area of philosophy of psychiatry. It has given us, as Austin would have anticipated, a more complete picture of the concepts which shape our understanding of Mrs Lazy's case and of psychopathological concepts generally. It has shown us that neither mind-only accounts of psychopathology, characteristic of some forms of anti-psychiatry, nor brain-only accounts, characteristic of the more triumphalist among biological psychiatrists, are sufficient. To have neglected Mrs Lazy's tumour would have been negligent. It would have been equally negligent, though, to have neglected her experience, her status as an autonomous agent, and her values. An adequate account of her case, therefore, and by extension of other less obviously brain-based cases of psychopathology, requires both. It requires the mental aspects of mind emphasised by antipsychiatry, and it requires the bodily aspects emphasised by biological psychiatry.

This is not a 'solution' to the mind-body problem, of course. In Austin's terms, it is no more than a way of getting started. But as Quinton anticipated, in the quote at the start of this chapter, it is a potentially fruitful way of getting started. As a basis for cross-disciplinary work between philosophy and psychiatry, the structure of experience and the nature of agency are already moving fast up the agenda of philosophy of mind. Several chapters in this book reflect this.

Psychopathology, I have suggested, providing as it does a bridge between moral and medical concepts, suggests that values, too, will soon be on the agenda of philosophy of mind. As Mrs Lazy's case shows, this will be good for psychiatry, both clinically and in neuroscience research; and it will be good for philosophy too. This is an area of cross-disciplinary work, then, in which, with a final echo of Austin, it is the "negative concept" which may wear the trousers [Austin, 1956/57]. It is the *disorders* of mind to which real people are subject which may turn out to be the sharpest philosophical probes into the nature of *mind.*

Acknowledgements

Parts of this chapter are adapted from section 2.3, *Introduction to the Philosophy of Mind and Mental Health Practice* of the *Distance Learning Course Book* for the Masters Course in *Philosophy, Ethics and Mental Health Practice*, Department of Philosophy, University of Warwick. I am grateful to Paul Sturdee and Tim Thornton, as my co-authors of the Course Book, for permission to reproduce the relevant sections here. The "Case of Mrs Lazy", as an article in The

Times newspaper, was spotted originally by Paul Sturdee. The "Map of Psychiatry" in the Figure appeared first in Fulford (1993b).

References

American Psychiatric Association (1994*) Diagnostic and statistical manual of mental disorders* (fourth edition). Washington, DC: American Psychiatric Association.

Austin, J. L. (1956-7) 'A plea for excuses. Proceedings of the Aristotelian' Society 57:1-30. Reprinted in White, A.R., ed. (1968) *The Philosophy of Action.* Oxford: Oxford University Press.

Bolton, D. (1998) 'Philosophy of Mind and Psychiatry'. *Current Opinion in Psychiatry,* 11, 563-566.

Bolton, D and Hill, J. (1996) *Mind, Meaning and Mental Disorder: the Nature of Causal Explanation in Psychology and Psychiatry.* Oxford: Oxford University Press.

Braude, S.E. (1991; also second edition, 1995) *First person plural: multiple personality and the philosophy of mind.* London: Routledge.

Braude, S.E. (1996) 'Multiple Personality and Moral Responsibility', *Philosophy, Psychiatry and Psychology*, 3, 37-54. Commentaries by Clark, S.R.L., pp. 55-58 and Shuman, D.W., pp. 59-60.

Campbell, J. (1994) *Past, Space, Self.* Cambridge, Mass: MIT Press.

Campbell, P. (1996) 'What we want from Crisis Services.' pp. 180-183, in Read, J. and Reynolds J., (eds.) *Speaking our Minds: an Anthology.* London: MacMillan Press Ltd.

Chadwick, R. F. (1994)' Kant, Thought Insertion and Mental Unity', *Philosophy, Psychiatry and Psychology*, 1, 105 - 114. Commentaries by Stephens, G.L. and Graham, G., pp. 115 - 116.

Clark, S.R.L. (1996) 'Minds, memes and multiples.' *Philosophy, Psychiatry and Psychology*, 3, 21-28. Commentaries by Bavidge, M. 29-30, and Sprigge, T. 31-36.

Fulford, K. W. M. 1989 (reprinted in paperback, 1995. Second edition due 1999) *Moral Theory and Medical Practice.* Cambridge: Cambridge University Press.

Fulford, K. W. M. 'Philosophy and Medicine: The Oxford Connection'. *British Journal of Psychiatry* 1990, 157:111-15.

Fulford K.W. M. (1991)' Evaluative Delusions: their Significance for Philosophy and Psychiatry', *British Journal of Psychiatry*, Volume 159, pp. 108-112, Supplement 14, Delusions and Awareness of Reality.

Fulford, K. W. M. (1993a) 'Mental illness and the mind-brain problem: delusion, belief and Searle's theory of intentionality'. *Theoretical*

Medicine; 14:181-94.
Fulford K. W. M. (1993b) 'Value, Action, Mental Illness and the Law'. pp. 279 - 310 in Shute S., Gardner J, and Horder J., eds. *Action and Value in Criminal Law.* Oxford: Oxford University Press.
Fulford, K.W.M. (1994) 'Closet logics: hidden conceptual elements in the DSM and ICD classifications of mental disorders'. Chapter 9 in Sadler, J.Z., Wiggins, O.P., Schwartz, M.A., eds. *Philosophical Perspectives on Psychiatric Diagnostic Classification.* Baltimore: Johns Hopkins University Press.
Fulford, K. W. M. (1998).'Philosophy and cross-cultural psychiatry'. Chapter 2 in Bhui, K. and Olajide, D., (eds.) *Studies in Cross-Cultural Psychiatry.* London: W.B. Saunders, Ltd.
Fulford, K. W. M., Smirnoff A.Y.U. and Snow. E. (1993). 'Concepts of disease and the abuse of psychiatry in the USSR'. *British Journal of Psychiatry* 162:801-10. (Reprinted 1996 in Medical Ethics, ed. R. S. Downie , volume in The International Research Library of Philosophy series, series ed. J. Skorupski. Aldershot, England: Dartmouth.)
Gindro, S., and Mordini, E. (1998) 'Ethical, Legal and Social Issues in Brain Research'. *Current Opinion in Psychiatry,* 11, 575-580.
Glover, J. (1988) I: *The Philosophy and Psychology of Personal Identity.* London: The Penguin Group.
Graham, G and Stephens, G. Lynn (1994) *Philosophical Psychopathology.* Cambridge, Mass: The MIT Press.
Hallen, B. And Sodipo, J. Olubi, (1997) *Knowledge, Belief and Witchcraft: Analytic Experiments in African Philosophy.* Stanford, California: Stanford University Press.
Hare, R.M. (1952) *The language of morals.* Oxford University Press.
Hare, R.M. (1963) 'Descriptivism'. *Proceedings of the British Academy* 49: 115-134. Reprinted in Hare, R.M. (1972) *Essays on the moral concepts.* London: The Macmillan Press Ltd.
Jackson, M. and Fulford, K. W. M. (1997) "Spiritual Experience and Psychopathology", *Philosophy, Psychiatry and Psychology,* 4, pp. 41-66 (Commentaries by Littlewood, R., Lu, F. G. et al, Sims, A. and Storr, A., with response by authors, pp. 67-90).
Jaspers K (1913a) 'Allgemeine Psychopathologi'. Berlin, Springer. In translation, Hoenig, J. and Hamilton M.W. (1963) *General Psychpathology* . Manchester: Manchester University Press.
Jaspers, K. (1913b) 'Causal and Meaningful Connexions Between Life History and Psychosis'. Chapter 5 in Hirsch, S.R. and Shepherd, M. eds. (1974) *Themes and Variations in European Psychiatry.* Bristol: John Wright and Sons Ltd.

Luntley, M. (1998) *Contemporary Philosophy of Thought*. Oxford: Blackwells.
McGinn, C. (1982) *The Character of Mind*. Oxford: Oxford University Press.
McGinn, C. (1993) 'Consciousness and Cosmology: Hyperdualism Ventilated' in Davies, M. and Humphreys, G.W., (eds.), *Consciousness: Psychological and Philosophical Essays*. Oxford: Blackwell.
Mishara, A.L., Parnas, J., and Naudin, J. (1998) 'Forging the links between phenomenology, cognitive neuroscience, and psychopathology: the emergence of a new discipline'. *Current Opinion in Psychiatry*, 11, pp.567-573.
Nordenfelt, L. (1987) *On the nature of health: an action-theoretic approach*. Dordrecht, Holland: D. Reidel Publishing Company.
Philpott, M.J. (1998) 'A phenomenology of Dyslexia: The Lived-Body, Ambiguity, and the Breakdown of Expression'. *Philosophy, Psychiatry and Psychology*, 5, 1-20. Commentaries by Komesaroff, P.A. and Wiltshire, J., pp. 21-24; Rippon, G., pp. 25-28; and Widdershovern, G.A.M., pp. 29-32. Response by author, pp. 33-36.
Quinton, A. (1985) 'Madness'. Chapter 2 in Griffiths, A.P., ed. *Philosophy and Practice*. Cambridge: Cambridge University Press.
Radden, J. (1996) *Divided Minds and Successive Selves: Ethical Issues in Disorders of Identity and Personality*, Cambridge, Mass: MIT Press.
Read, J. (1996) 'What we want from mental health services'. pp. 175-179 in Read, J. and Reynolds, J., eds. *Speaking our Minds: an Anthology*. London: MacMillan Press Ltd.
Re C. (adult: refusal of medical treatment), (1994) 1 All ER 819.
Roth, M. and Kroll, J. (1986) *The Reality of Mental Illness*. Cambridge University Press.
Sadler, J.S. and Agich, G.J. (1995) 'Diseases, Functions, Values, and Philosophy, Psychiatry and Psychopathy Psychiatric Classification'. *Philosophy, Psychiatry, and Psychology*, 2, 219 – 232.
Shorter, E. (1997) *A History of Psychiatry*, New York: John Wiley and Sons.
Stephens, G.L. and Graham, G. (1994) 'Self-Consciousness, Mental Agency and Psychopathology'. *Philosophy, Psychiatry and Psychology*, 1, 1 - 10. (Commentary by Wiggins, O. P., pp. 11-12.)
Szasz, T.S. (1960) *The myth of mental illness*. American Psychologist, 15: 113-118.
Toulmin, S. (1980) 'Agent and patient in psychiatry'. *International*

Journal of Law and Psychiatry, 3, pp.267-78. Wakefield, J.C. (1995) 'Dysfunction as a Value-Free Concept: a Reply to Sadler and Agich'. *Philosophy, Psychiatry, and Psychology*, 2, 233 – 246.

Warnock, G.J. (1989) *J L Austin.* London: Routledge.

Wilkes, K.V. (1988) *Real People: Personal Identity Without Thought Experiments.* Oxford: Clarendon Press.

Wing, J.K., Cooper, J.E. and Sartorius, N. (1974) *Measurement and classification of psychiatric symptoms.* Cambridge University Press.

World Health Organisation (1992) *The ICD-10 Classification of Mental and Behavioural Disorders: Clinical Descriptions and Diagnostic Guidelines.* Geneva: World Health Organisation.

5 Mental Content and the Myth of Problems in Living

MARTIN JOHNSTON

Introduction

Traditional 'debates' concerning the nature of mental disorder have tended to become polarised around two conflicting approaches: those which identify mental disorder as the manifestation of particular underlying physical states and processes, and those which seek to provide translations or reconstructions of talk about mental disorder into talk about socialisation, behaviour, labelling and the like. (Of course this characterisation is too general; in particular it ignores the realist/nominalist debate (Kendell, 1991) within medical psychiatry, but it should prove sufficient for the particular purposes of this chapter.) Such polarisation of opinion has done little in terms of providing a useful foundation for constructive discussion, as Cavadino (1989) points out, the situation is one where members of opposing camps refuse to acknowledge the legitimacy of the other's key terms and concepts, rendering attempts to engage in meaningful dialogue futile. The image of two competing forces shouting at one another across an unbridgeable chasm is particularly relevant here. That neither pole can clearly be said to have won the day is indicative of particular inadequacies and/or problems with completeness associated with the positions at either pole. My basic thesis is that psychopathic condition often involves a significant lack of certain reactive attitudes and that this has interesting moral implications for our treatment of psychopaths. But I do not want to overstate the case, since there are probably people with marked psychopathic traits who do entertain at least some of these attitudes. We should remember that psychopathy, like moral responsibility, probably admits of degree; and we should bear in mind that even if a marked absence of at least some of these attitudes in a frequent hallmark of psychopathy, it need not be a necessary or sufficient condition for it.

It is well beyond the scope of this chapter to address all such inadequacies and problems, however, what I hope to show is that bridge building is a viable project, and whilst I may not be able to provide the finished bridge, it is possible to identify particular foundations upon which such a bridge has the potential to be secure. In order to do this a degree of simplification is required. In what follows I propose to consider the work of Thomas Szasz as representative of the antipsychiatry movement, and a realist version of the medical model.

The models

The crux of the realist conception of mental disorder is that such disorder is accurately described as illness. That is, the range of phenomena associated with mental disorder are properly identified as the consequences of underlying disease or impairment at the physical level. The degree of confidence with which proponents of this view talk of the possibility of identifying physical causes for all such phenomena varies, but in spite of this the fundamental tenet remains. In philosophical terms it appears that some version of the mind/brain identity thesis is implicit in such a view, though of course some strained version of dualism may remain, but this is unlikely to prove to be particularly attractive to contemporary psychiatrists.

By way of stark contrast, Szasz (1961) asserts that there is no such thing as mental illness; what perhaps once proved to be a useful theoretical construct has come to be seen as fact, a state of affairs which has led to major violations of rights to liberty over the years. The core of Szasz's view is that psychiatric diagnosis is an essentially evaluative project, which masquerades as scientific practice, leading to a misclassification of "problems in living" as mental illness. In particular he points to the failure on the part of medical psychiatry to provide sufficient evidence in terms of identifying the physical causes of 'mental illness' (Szasz, 1963), as grounds for supporting his view. Where such causal foundations have been identified - for example the discovery that syphilis infection led to general paralysis of the insane - Szasz argues that such conditions are more accurately described as diseases of the brain. But his claims go much further than this, central to his thesis is the view that mental illness concepts are applied to behaviour not physical states (Szasz, 1990), and hence any reductive project in physical terms is misguided. In as much as this is an accurate depiction of Szasz's view, it is difficult to classify his position in the terminology of standard philosophy of mind other than perhaps identifying a fairly strong behaviourist component; nevertheless we can clearly see that he is not a reductive materialist. So much then for the chasm; what of the bridge?

Philosophy of mind and psychiatry

I have already alluded to the philosophical assumptions underlying each of the approaches, although in the case of Szasz this has been only a negative characterisation, clearly some further development is required. In order to achieve this I would like to consider the impact of recent developments in philosophy of mind concerning the nature of mental content, in particular the internalism v. externalism debate. A neat encapsulation of these two theses is provided by McGinn:

"Recent philosophy of mind has been much exercised with the question whether mental states are 'in the head'. *Internalism* is the thesis that they are; *externalism* is the thesis that they are not." (McGinn, 1991, p.1.) But of course there is more to the issue than this. McGinn goes on to say:

"Externalism (like internalism) is best construed as a thesis about the *individuation* of mental states: a thesis, that is, about the existence and identity conditions of mental states. It places conditions on the existence of a mental state in a possible situation, and it tells us what kinds of changes preserve the identity of a mental state - these being a matter of relations to the environment. The environment is thus held to be constitutive of the very nature of mental states, determining what they *are*." (McGinn, p.3.)

Much of the impetus for the formulation of externalism stems from responses to Putnam's claims concerning meaning (Putnam, 1980, pp215-271) - in particular the meaning of natural kind terms - with their use of the celebrated Twin Earth examples, which lead to the famous conclusion: "Cut the pie any way you like, 'meanings' just ain't in the *head*!" (p227) Externalism then involves an implicit realism concerning the world, and emphasises the importance of objects and kinds of substance in the environment in the delineation of mental states.

Internalism, on the other hand, rests on the assumption of what McCulloch refers to as the "self-containedness thesis" (McCulloch, 1995), that is, the view that the mind could exist as it is irrespective of any environmental conditions. Such methodological solipsism underpins much of the dominant tradition in recent philosophy of mind generally, and philosophy of psychology in particular; at least following the demise of behaviourism. But it is precisely this assumption which is put to the test by Putnam's claims, and is arguably found wanting. Be that as it may, there is much in the externalism/internalism debate which can inform the present discussion, and it is to such issues that we now turn.

On this account the realist version of the medical model is compatible with, but does not entail, internalism, taking as it does the underlying neurophysiological states as the basis of the phenomena associated with mental disorder. In these terms a brain in a vat could be schizophrenic for example, though whether such a state of affairs could pertain is a fundamental issue for an adequate philosophy of psychiatry. Szasz's account on the other hand is much more difficult to classify in these terms. In part this is due to his primary concern being with third person ascriptions of psychiatric diagnostic categories; further his account of 'problems in living' is lacking in causal detail. Other than general remarks concerning liberty, which appear to involve an implicit conception of free will, we are left very much in the dark with regard to Szasz's positive conception of the nature of mind. Again we shall deal with a negative conception of Szasz's philosophical roots.

On one reading at least, Szasz is not an internalist in as much as he denies the importance of underlying disordered physical states to the appearance of symptoms of mental disorder, but of course this does not of itself exhaust the possible criteria for being an internalist. Whether this makes him an externalist is a question we shall leave unanswered for the moment. But it is in the pursuit of an answer to this question that we can identify a range of issues which I hope will provide the foundations identified earlier. In order to this I propose to consider only a limited number of psychotic symptoms, principally delusions and hallucinations.

Mental content and psychotic symptoms

Delusions

There is no dispute concerning the existence of a range of phenomena associated with mental disorder. People experience hallucinations, hold delusional beliefs, experience levels of fear disproportionate to the known level of threat presented and the like, the issues for debate concern the origins and true natures of such phenomena. Dealing first with delusions, we can set up the difference between Szasz and the medical model as follows. Classically medical definitions of delusions refer to fixed, false beliefs not open to rational persuasion, or explicable in terms of cultural influences or socialisation processes. Szasz makes the following points:

> We speak of mental symptoms, on the other hand, when we refer to a patient's communications about himself, others and the world about him. He might state that he is Napoleon or that he is being persecuted by the Communists. These would be considered mental symptoms *only* if the observer believed that the patient was *not* Napoleon or that he was *not* being persecuted by the Communists. (Szasz, 1965, p.13)

We shall initially deal with the issue of the falsity of a belief as indicative of its delusional status. The implicit realism associated with externalism offers the possibility of providing criteria for the proper identification of false beliefs - of course being a realist about the world is not the exclusive prerogative of the externalist - but arguably this is limited. Putnam's claims are strongest in reference to natural kind terms, and though some may, clearly not all delusional, or indeed false, beliefs concern natural kinds. In a similar vein it is difficult to accurately depict where Szasz's position lies. The statement above gives very strong hints towards subjectivism which seems to direct Szasz towards the internalist camp, this may be mistaken, but that is a consequence of the absence of a positive account of the nature of mind in his writing.

More important are the claims made concerning the nature of the observer's beliefs. Szasz appears to suggest that the identification of a false belief rests upon essentially arbitrary grounds. Even when dealing with more complex beliefs, like the examples given by Szasz, whilst we may not be able to exploit the full power of realism concerning natural kinds, we are still entitled to talk of warrant in relation to beliefs. Again we can turn to Putnam (1992, pp. 3-29) who establishes criteria by which we can identify standards in order to apply notions of better and worse to beliefs about the world. The most important aspect of which is that such notions are not solely determined by communal agreement. In general this leaves us with a situation where we can talk clearly in some circumstances of the truth and falsity of beliefs, and in others of degrees of warrant.

Of course not all false beliefs are delusional, nor indeed need all delusional beliefs be false, there is room for genuine error or unwarrantable correctness so the base from which we identify delusional beliefs has to be expanded. A key feature of Szasz's view here is the use of the word 'only'. I can very well believe that the person before me is Napleon, whilst considering his claims that he is Napoleon to be delusion. To make this clear, imagine that Napoleon presents in the consulting room with profound amnesia, his assertion that he is Napoleon rests on two counts, that he is small, and that he is French. I on the other hand have a much broader base upon which to make my assertion that he is Napoleon stemming from the fact that I was his field surgeon throughout his many campaigns. Essentially we are dealing with the issue of the rationality of beliefs. In the above case I challenge Napoleon's belief that he is Napoleon not on the grounds of the truth or falsity of that belief, but rather of the sufficiency of the conditions which render it warranted. We can develop this idea further with reference to an example from Fulford (1995), where an apparently paradoxical situation arises when a patient is committed for psychiatric treatment partly on the grounds of the expression of the belief that he is mad.

Taking the issue of truth and falsity, which perhaps is the origin of apparent paradox in this case, a first attempt to formalise the problem might look something like this:

X (the patient) believes "X is mad" – q
Y (the psychiatrist) believes not q therefore q

Were this to be an accurate formalisation then there is serious cause for alarm, but of course it falls dramatically short of so being.
The inaccuracy here rests on the mistaken ascription of the belief 'not q' to the psychiatrist.
A more accurate representation requires a further premise.
If X has delusional beliefs then X is mad
or
If p then q

In which case the psychiatrist's reasoning is straightforward:
If p then q
p
Therefore q

The case illustrates the dangers in taking falsity to be the defining characteristic of delusions. What the psychiatrist here needs is an alternative set of defining characteristics for delusions. The veracity of beliefs like 'I am mad', 'My eyes are dead', 'I am Napoleon', is not the significant issue. In many respects this amounts to saying that the 'truth' of the belief drops out. The significant issue becomes one of warrant or justification. There is some sense in which falsity can come to be seen as a shorthand for warrant. When someone holds a false belief it is, perhaps, difficult to imagine sufficient grounds or warrant for that belief, but not impossible, this may explain the inclusion of the absence of cultural influences in standard medical definitions of delusions.

Returning to the original case then, apparent difficulties still remain even though we now extend the patient's reasoning to parallel the psychiatrist's:
X's belief then takes the form of a conditional.
If p then q, where p is used to identify the grounds for X's belief.
Perhaps alarmingly this appears identical to the psychiatrist, of course it is not because p is not identical in both cases. Interestingly there is a

sense in which talk of truth and falsity re-enters here. It is the truth or falsity of 'If p then q' which is at issue. Cashing in p and q, making no distinction between first and third person ascription, we could get something like this:

Psychiatrist
If X has delusional beliefs then X is mad
X has delusional beliefs
X is mad

Patient
If X has brown hair then X is mad
X has brown hair
X is mad

In this case the identification of a particular belief as false, though present, is not the most significant feature, since what we should be more concerned about are the reasons why the patient believes the first premise of his argument.

Now I do not claim to have established definitively a complete account of the nature of delusions, and indeed the absence of a complete and general account of the grounds for accepting a persuasive argument or set of arguments may cause one to lose heart, but once again it does not follow from this that no adequate account can be given in particular cases. And indeed we can point to systems in formal logic which go some way towards specifying rules of inference and reasoning. All of which points to the possibility of identifying flaws in the construction of beliefs, which can then be utilised as further criteria in the identification of delusions. This then lends weight to a rejection of Szasz's claims concerning the apparent arbitrariness of the observer's opinion regarding the truth or falsity of the patient's beliefs.

Where Szasz appears to be on firmer ground is when dealing with the role of cultural influences on belief. A belief is not delusional in these terms so long as it is shared by others. It is this type of criterion which provides Szasz with substantial ammunition, by enlisting the support of others one becomes a pressure group rather than a case for psychiatric referral. But while such an approach to delusion beliefs may, in a number of cases, prove politically expedient, it is philosophically unsatisfactory in terms of characterising delusions since it is based upon a fairly arbitrary foundation. From what has gone before, the possibility of collective adherence to unwarranted beliefs has not been ruled out, but consensus is not warrant.

Hallucinations

We turn now to an account of hallucinations. In this case the error in the perceptual experience is identified by reference to the absence of any appropriate external stimulus, and again if we are prepared to make certain realist commitments then, in most cases, it is a relatively straightforward matter to identify when this is the case. It is a criterion of the veracity of my perception of a voice instructing me to kill myself that there be an external source of that voice. Again a number of possible error conditions enter the scene, but once more this should not lead us to the conclusion that it is never possible to distinguish between genuine and hallucinatory perceptions. If this were the case then Macbeth's question concerning the dagger simply wouldn't make sense. But again the issue is not one purely of the truth or falsity of the actual experience. If we take belief formation to be the end product of perception, then what we are dealing with here are atypical sources of belief, that is, the beliefs associated with hallucinations are not caused in the right sorts of way. A drug induced perception of the contents of a blacked out room may correspond exactly to the actual relative distributions of objects in that room, but nonetheless remains hallucinatory since it is not caused in the appropriate way.

It is this notion of the causes of hallucinatory experiences which presents Szasz with his greatest challenge. Whilst one can recognise a variety of responses to the pressures of modern life, which may accurately be described as problems in living, that these should become manifest in the form of hallucinatory experiences remains problematic. A crucial point here is that there appears to be something projective about hallucinations, in terms of the medical model it is plausible to suggest that such projections are the result of disordered brain function, as would be the case where the influence of drugs was a contributing factor for example, but Szasz does not appear to have any access to such an explanation. (Except of course where his point concerning the proper identification of mental illness as illness of the brain holds.) His apparent rejection of internalism leaves him with a very sticky problem indeed. This still leaves the question of the charaterisation of Szasz's view in internalist/externalist terms unanswered, but nonetheless an important avenue for exploration is opened up.

Internalism, externalism and the philosophy of psychiatry

The discussion of the nature of phenomena such as delusions and hallucinations is primarily a discussion of the nature of particular mental states and part of that discussion has to be concerned with the individuation of those states. The identification of a belief as delusional, or of a perception as hallucinatory, in many instances is clearly a complicated process, but much will depend upon where we locate the content of those states. There is, for example, a clear initial appeal in locating the content of psychotic symptoms 'in the head' of the individual concerned, but this would be to grossly oversimplify matters. Indeed it would perhaps be legitimate to describe Szasz's account as highlighting some the inadequacies associated with taking a purely internalist view of mental illness, and he is right to do so, but this does not make him an externalist. It is my contention that the attempts to provide an adequate philosophy of psychiatry, represented by the poles of opinion discussed in this paper, founder because of a failure to come to terms with the range of issues raised by the internalism/externalism debate.

What is at issue is the full complexity of the relationship between mind and world, and this becomes even more apparent when we move away from the relatively secure ground of psychotic symptoms. A yet broader picture of the difficulties can be obtained if we consider psychopathy. In many respects the difficulty here lies in the fact that we are not dealing with specific beliefs and perceptions, but rather with something more like a general attitude towards the world. Classical descriptions of psychopathy tend to highlight features such as an absence of empathy and an essentially amoral approach to the world, neither of which initially fit comfortably with the idea of particular mental states. Nevertheless, many of the central concerns related to the definition of psychopathy can be addressed in terms of internalism and externalism. If we are to decide that a characteristic feature like the absence of empathy is a genuine symptom of mental disorder, then we must be able to separate this from cases of genuine error and deliberate deception, as I have attempted to do in the cases of delusional beliefs and hallucinations - though not in anything like a complete sense. There may even be a sense in which we could translate talk of the absence of empathy into talk of an albeit elaborate delusory belief system about the nature of others. Amorality again admits of definition in terms of complex belief systems, but in both cases there is clearly a story which has to be told concerning the formation of beliefs. It is in addressing this issue - not something which I propose to deal with here - that the full detail of understanding the interaction of the mind and world comes to the fore. What does seem initially implausible is that an entirely internalist account of mind would prove sufficient.

But the preceding account of delusions and hallucinations appears to involve many internalist claims, with regard to the origins of psychotic symptoms, in the absence of competing causal claims there does seem to be something very much 'in the head' about such phenomena, this appears somewhat confusing at first sight. It is important to note however, that a commitment to externalism does not require that we deny the existence of accompanying neurophysiological states, as McCulloch points out (1985). In addition McGinn (1991) distinguishes between weak and strong versions of externalism, the former allowing for the possibility of mental states having essentially projective features which appear necessary to a convincing account of the nature of psychotic symptoms. However there is clearly a substantial amount of further work to be done, and I would suggest that much of this consist in the evaluation of the implications of externalism for a philosophy of psychiatry. In many respects I may have failed in my attempt to provide foundations for the future, but at least I think that I have pointed to where it may be most appropriate to start the survey.

Conclusion

If my account thus far is at all plausible then what begins to emerge is the need for an account of delusions and hallucinations which incorporates recent developments in the philosophy of mind. On the basis of this it should prove possible to move from facts concerning the existence of delusions and hallucinations to facts concerning their natures. The significance of this in relation to offering a critique of Szasz's account is central. To account for the differences between genuine perceptions and hallucinations, delusional and non-delusional beliefs, it appears necessary to point to features of the individual subject. This need not involve an endorsement of some explanation couched purely in terms of the physical characteristics of the subject's central nervous system, but then nor does it rule it out. What is more seriously open to challenge is the view that such experiences are appropriately described as problems in living, except in the trivial sense that anyone having such experiences will no doubt have problems in living. In a particular case where the factual basis of a delusion or hallucination can be established, then we have removed the value aspect of the judgement "X is a mental symptom", in such cases we are no longer dealing with arbitrary constructions based on particular socially determined points of view, or indeed with myths. Indeed if there are any myths at work it is when the facts of delusions and hallucinations are assigned to the category of "problems in living".

References

Cavadino, M. (1989), *Mental Health Law in Context: Doctors Orders.* Aldershot: Dartmouth.

Fulford, K.W.M. (1995), *Moral Theory and Medical Practice.* Cambridge: Cambridge University Press.

Kendell, R.E. (1991), 'The Major Functional Psychoses: are they independent entities or part of a Continuum? Philosophical and conceptual issues underlying the debate', in Kerr, A. and McClelland, H. eds., *Concepts of Mental Disorder: A Continuing debate.* London: Gaskell.

McGinn, C. (1991), *Mental Content.* Oxford: Blackwell.

Putnam, H. (1980), 'The Meaning of 'Meaning'', in *Mind, Language and Reality: Philosophical Papers*, Volume 2. Cambridge: Cambridge University Press.

Putnam, H. (1992), 'Realism with a Human Face'; in Conant, J. ed. (1992), *Realism with a Human Face*. Boston: Harvard University Press.

Szasz, T. (1961), *The Myth of Mental Illness*. New York: Hoeber-Harper.

Szasz, T. (1963), *Law, Liberty and Psychiatry*. London: Routledge and Kegan-Paul.

Szasz, T. (1990), 'Law and Psychiatry: the problems that will not go away'. *Journal of Mind and Behavour*, 11, No 4.

6 The Concept of Mental Injury

STEPHEN WILKINSON

Introduction

In a previous paper, I argued that conditions such as normal grief are mental maladies: i.e. states of "mental unhealth". (Wilkinson 1997) This paper aims to deal with some of the more general theoretical implications of adopting this view of grief. I start by very briefly summarising my reasons for viewing normal grief as a mental malady and then attempt to sketch a more general account of the concept of *mental injury*. Finally, I address a number of possible objections to this account.

The theoretical backdrop to the previous paper was my broad support for Clouser, Culver and Gert's account of maladies (both mental and physical). Their theory is neatly summed up by the following quotations. They first introduce the general term "malady":

> As we use the term, "malady" refers to that which all the other disease words have in common: "injury", "illness", "sickness", "disease", "trauma", "wound", "disorder", "lesion", "allergy", "headache", "syndrome", and so on.
> (Clouser, Culver and Gert, 1997, p177)

And then proceed to define it as follows:

> ... Individuals have a malady if and only if they have a condition, other than their rational beliefs and desires, such that they are incurring, or are at a significantly increased risk of incurring, a harm or evil (death, pain, disability, loss of

> freedom, or loss of pleasure) in the absence of a distinct sustaining cause. (Clouser, Culver and Gert, 1997, p. 190)

My argument was simple in structure. Normal grief necessarily involves mental pain, does not consist wholly of rational beliefs and desires, and does not usually have a distinct sustaining cause. Therefore, it meets Clouser, Culver and Gert's criterion for being a malady, a criterion which I accept. Interestingly, Culver and Gert (1982, p96) have argued that normal grief is *not* a malady because (on their view) it has a distinct sustaining cause (the loss of a loved one). But in 'Is Grief a Mental Malady?' I spend a considerable amount of time refuting this claim and, thereby, demonstrating that their theory really *does* imply that normal grief is a mental malady.

The "Intuitive" View That (Normal) Grief Is Not a Disease

Many people are very hostile to classifying normal grief as a mental malady. To say that grievers are "mentally ill" or suffering from "a disease" seems to them like too strong a claim to make. And several people have made comments like the following to me:

> Of course, (normal) grievers are suffering and have had a misfortune, but there's nothing wrong *with their health*. Their problem isn't mental *illness*, but rather the pain arising from a tragic *event* or *situation*.

There is certainly *some* truth in this sort of remark, although I do not believe that it gives us sufficient reason not to classify normal grief as a malady. What is right about the remark is the idea that there is some feature of the main cause of normal grief (eg. the loss of a loved one) which makes us rightly reluctant to call it a disease or illness.

Physical Injury and Mental Injury: an analogy

Consider a fairly standard case in which someone who is otherwise very fit and healthy receives a minor sports injury, say, a sprained ankle. It would be very odd to say that such a person was *diseased* and similarly odd, although much less so, to say that she was *ill*. What we want to say of such a person is just that they are *injured* (although if the injury were of a more serious nature then words such as "disability" and "illness" would start to look more appropriate).

Shortly, I shall explore in more detail the concept of injury. But for the time being let me offer one tentative reason for our *not* wishing to say that our sports injury victim is diseased. It is that the cause of the malady in question is a one-off event which (in some as yet unspecified sense) occurred outside the person.

It is my contention that it is helpful to think about normal grief in a similar way. We are rightly reluctant to classify it as a *disease* or *mental illness* because it is caused by a one-off event which (again, in some as yet unspecified sense) was external to the person grieving. But the difference between the physical and the mental case is that, whereas for physical health we are used to operating with a distinction between injury and disease, this is much less common for mental health. Hence, given that there is no widely accepted category "mental injury" into which to put normal grief, we take our reasons for not classifying it as a disease to be reasons for not classifying it as a malady at all.

II Physical Injury

As far as possible, we should attempt to construct a *unified* account of health concepts, especially with respect to mental and physical health: i.e. we should aim to construct health concepts which are applicable to both mental and physical conditions. Of course, it is not possible in advance of philosophical (and, in some cases, clinical) investigation to tell whether this is an aim which is achievable and it may turn out that mental and physical health concepts are importantly different from one another. However, the *default* assumption should be that physical and mental health concepts are at least very similar. Hence, I start my enquiry by analysing the concept of physical injury, which I take to be less controversial and problematic than that of mental injury.

The first point to make is that the distinction between physical injury and disease is itself, at best, vague. Reznek provides an effective account of the reasons for this:

> Take the distinction between injury and disease - the natures of diseases are not of a different type from the natures of injuries. For example, if a man is savaged by a lion, we do not consider that he has acquired a disease. Similarly, if a man is devoured by killer ants, we still do not classify this biological interaction as a disease. However, the interaction with yet smaller organisms (like fungi, bacteria, or viruses), and the interaction with organisms that are not visible (like gastrointestinal worms) *are* considered to be diseases. Yet there do not seem to be any theoretically important differences between the extremes - all are interactions with other organisms where man is adversely affected, and just how big or visible the organism is seems theoretically unimportant. (Reznek 1987, p68)

Insofar as there is a workable distinction between (physical) injury and disease, though, it is dependent on certain properties of the *causes* of the relevant malady. As Reznek suggests, it seems that maladies get classified as injuries when their causes are large, visible, unmysterious and external. However, can such ideas really form the basis of an account of injury?

Of the four properties just mentioned, it seems that *externality* is the one best placed to provide a distinction between injury and other maladies and I shall now explain and defend the following definition of injury, based on the idea of externality:

The Externality Account of Injury

X is an injury if and only if:

(a) it is a malady; and,
(b) its main immediate cause is *not* an internal process.

Obviously, (a) is a necessary condition, since injury is one *type* of malady. So the questions that need to be addressed are:

(i) is (b) also necessary?
(ii) are (a) and (b) jointly sufficient?

Before proceeding to test the externality account against cases, though, I should say something about why externality was chosen ahead of largeness, visibility and unmysteriousness. Visibility and unmysteriousness were rejected chiefly because they relativise to too great an extent the concept of injury to our cognitive and perceptual powers. If we used these as criteria we would, for example, be committed to saying that if humans found the relationship between being hit by a high-speed train and damage to one's health utterly mysterious (because perhaps we had a peculiar cognitive "blind-spot" about the effects of trains) then train crashes would cause (for example) *diseases* rather than injuries.

Similarly, we would be committed to saying that if our eyesight had been better, then various bacterial and fungal infections would have caused injury rather than disease. Such relativisation to our cognitive/perceptual powers is both counter-intuitive and would make the distinction between injury and other maladies completely arbitrary and of little use for either theory or practice.

Although using size as a criterion would not be dogged by quite the same difficulty (size not being relative to our cognitive and perceptual capabilities) problems would arise when we attempted to set the appropriate size threshold. What reason could there be to prefer one size threshold, to another? In fact, it seems that insofar as a size threshold does figure in the ordinary concept of injury, it is based on visibility. But if we based our size threshold on visibility, then we would once again be relativising the concept of injury to how good our eyes are. Hence, a size criterion should be rejected.

Externality as a criterion has two distinct advantages. First, it is less arbitrary and less dependent on our cognitive and perceptual capabilities than the other candidates, since although even for externality there will be tricky borderline cases, there is at least *usually* some fact of the matter as to whether some process is internal to the person or not. Second, externality can go a long way towards explaining why the other three candidates do apparently figure in the everyday concept of injury. For if injuries have external things as their main causes, then it is hardly surprising that these are going to bigger, more visible and less mysterious than the causes of other maladies.

The internal processes which cause other maladies will almost always be invisible (to the ordinary unaided observer) and are therefore much more likely to be mysterious (although they needn't be). Similarly larger objects are, just for practical reasons, much less likely to figure in internal bodily processes (although again I think this is more a matter of probability than necessity). So externality is to be preferred *both* because the other candidates face serious problems that it does not *and* because it can go some way towards accommodating and explaining any intuitive appeal that the other candidates have.

Easy Cases for the Externality Account

Having outlined briefly my reasons for preferring the externality account, it will be useful now to see how it might apply to actual cases, starting with those for which it seems unproblematically to work well. Consider, for example, the following injuries:

1. breaking my leg in a football accident
2. burning myself on a kitchen hot plate
3. receiving gunshot wounds

And assume also that they had the following causes:

(a) another player stood on my leg
(b) I placed my hand on the hotplate
(c) someone shot me

All of these, I assume, are injuries and, what is more, they seem to fit perfectly with the externality account. More specifically, what seems to make it right to classify these conditions as injuries rather than diseases is that their main immediate causes - (a), (b), and (c) - are not internal processes. Rather, they are events which are external to me.

Hard Cases for the Externality Account

The externality account does not in every case seem to work so well, though, and in this section I shall consider two kinds of problem case: cases in which injuries are caused by diseases, and 'internal injuries'.

The first problem is that some injuries, it seems, are caused by diseases (which are internal to the person). For example, what if I break my leg and the cause is that I have a *brittle bone disorder*, such that the slightest knock will cause a break?

If it is assumed both (a) that the brittle bone disorder consists of *internal* processes and states and (b) that the brittle bone disorder is the main immediate cause of the break, then the externality account apparently leads to the conclusion that the broken leg is not in this case an injury. This is problematically counter-intuitive. For *this* broken leg seems to be just as much an injury as *any other* broken leg and, furthermore, one may well want to think of brittle bone disorders precisely as *dispositions to be injured* by normal contact with the environment.

The best way for the externality account to deal with such cases is by arguing that, although the brittle bone disorder is indeed a cause of the break, it is not an *immediate* cause, since only events can be *immediate* causes (in the sense of 'immediate cause' intended by the account) whereas the brittle bone disorder is a *disposition* rather than an event. By dealing with the case in this way, the externality account allows us both to classify the break as an injury and to allow that it is nevertheless a *symptom* of the bone disorder, since the causal relevance of the disorder is not called into question: i.e the disorder *is* a cause, but not an *immediate* one.

The second problem case is internal injuries. For if there are such things as *internal* injuries, clearly this may pose problems for an account which seeks to define 'injury' in terms of *externality*. The expression 'internal injuries' normally refers to one of two distinct (though, in practice, related) types of condition. The first are conditions where the injured body part is an internal organ. The second are those where the injurious event (the event which causes the injury) takes place inside the body - for example, if someone were to swallow a sharp object, or a small explosive device.

Internal injuries of the first type pose no *special* problem for the externality account and this should hardly be surprising given that *all* injured body parts are, in some sense, internal to the person. The reason why there is no special problem here is that the externality account takes the externality of the *causes* of the injury to be the relevant feature, not the externality of *the injury itself*. In other words, the claim is not that injuries are external, but that their immediate causes are. Hence, provided that the immediate cause of damage to my kidney (for example) is external, then it is an *injured* kidney. And to call such an injury 'internal' is just to signify that the injured part is a 'central' organ, as opposed to some more 'peripheral' body part, such as a finger.

Internal injuries of the second type are more problematic, since here the injurious event does take place within the body. Take, for instance the hypothetical case in which someone swallows a small time bomb which later explodes. Here, the immediate cause of any bodily damage is the explosion. So the problem for the externality account is that both of the following seem to be true:

(a) the main immediate cause of the bodily damage was an event which occurred *inside* the body;

(b) the bodily damage is an injury.

If both (a) and (b) are true then this case provides a powerful counter-example to the externality account.

The best way for the externality account to deal with this case is by arguing that although, *in one sense*, the injurious event is internal, it is not internal *in the relevant sense*. Under one construal, 'internal' just means *inside what is normally taken to be the outer boundary of the body* (i.e. the skin). And under this construal, the bomb and the explosion are, of course, internal. However, 'internal' could also be taken to mean something slightly more complex. Under this second (more complex) construal, things are genuinely internal to the body only if they have been, so to speak, only *internalised*: if they have engaged causally with the body's mechanisms and have interacted with it on what we might loosely call the 'micro-level'.

To illustrate the difference between these two interpretations of 'internal', consider the difference between swallowing an ordinary piece of food and swallowing a small ball of gold. In both cases, the object becomes internal (in the first sense) as soon as it is swallowed, since it is immediately inside the body's outer boundary. However, while it is likely that the piece of food will become *internalised* (through digestion etc.) this probably will not be the case for the ball of gold (assuming that it doesn't interact bio-chemically with the body and simply 'passes through' the digestive system). Hence, we might say of this case that whereas the food is (or becomes) internal, *in the second sense of internal*, the gold is not.

If the food contained a bacterial infection which caused a malady, we would *not* call this an injury, but rather an illness or a disease or poisoning. But if the gold formed a sharp object rather than a smooth ball and this caused internal lacerations, we may well want to classify this as an *internal injury*. The complex concept of internality suggested above (combined with the externality account of injury) goes a long way towards explaining and accommodating our differing intuitions about the classification of these cases. The immediate causes of the food poisoning are internal, since they consist of 'micro-level' interactions between the food and the body. But the immediate cause of the lacerations is the motion of an object which although inside the body is *not* internal in the relevant sense (i.e. *internalised*). Hence, the externality account achieves the desired 'intuitive' results.

Although, in this way, the externality account can be made to produce intuitive results when applied to hypothetical cases of 'internal injury', these cases do raise two more general theoretical issues, which need to be mentioned before commencing the discussion of mental injury.

The first is that we are reminded that the distinction between injury and other maladies is (as was suggested earlier) inevitably vague, one of the sources of that vagueness being the vagueness of the distinction between those events or objects that are internal (in the relevant sense) and those that are not. In other words, there will inevitably be some borderline cases in which it is just not possible to judge whether or not a particular thing has become internalised or not.

The second is that size may, after all, have some role to play in determining the distinction between physical injury and other physical maladies, since it has a role to play in determining the (relevant) distinction between internal and external. This is because, as was suggested above, one important part of something becoming *internalised* is how it interacts with the body at a 'micro-level'; and, of course, the distinction between micro and other-level interactions looks like a distinction based on size.

The position here is that size does, indeed, have an *indirect* role in determining which maladies are injuries, although it is not the crude role that was discussed and rejected earlier. It's role is as follows. The size of the objects that cause a given malady is (at least *in principle*) irrelevant to the question of whether that malady is an injury or not. What is relevant is whether (all or part of) the object becomes *internalised*. This is principally a matter of the *level* on which the object interacts with the body ('micro' or other) and questions of *level* are closely related to questions of size and scale. Hence, size does have a role to play because of its relation to different levels of physical interaction. However, there are (in principle) no constraints on the size of the objects which causes injuries, since it is possible for large objects (or parts thereof) to interact with bodies on a micro-level and, conversely, possible for very small objects to fail to do so, if they are appropriately inert.

III Mental Injury

Interestingly, Flew in his 'Disease and Mental Disease' (1981, p434) mentions in passing the fact that the *Royal Commission on the Law relating to Mental Illness and Mental Deficiency* found no "merit in any mental analogue of the distinction between [physical] wounds and diseases". In this section, I aim to cast some doubt on the Royal Commission's view and shall argue that the distinction between *mental* injuries (or wounds) and *mental* diseases is just as sustainable as that between *physical* injuries (or wounds) and *physical* diseases.

The Definition of "Mental Injuries"?

The view of mental injuries which I shall propose and go some way towards defending in the remaining part of this paper is that mental injuries are those mental maladies which do *not* have as their main immediate causes processes and states which are internal to the person. The account of mental injury offered is therefore structurally very similar to the externality account of physical injury just discussed and (for reasons suggested near the beginning of this paper) I take this to be one of its major theoretical advantages.

Internal and External

One advantage of the externality account of *physical injury* is that, in spite of some of the complications discussed earlier, the distinction between external and internal causes remains reasonably clear: not least because it is a distinction that can be understood, for the most part, in purely spatial terms. However, things seem less straightforward when talking about the internality or externality of mental states. Before proceeding, then, it is important to say briefly something about what the internal/external distinction means when it is applied to mental health.

For the purposes of defining mental injury a cause is internal *if and only if it is one of the person's mental states*. Obviously, for those who believe that mental states are identical with internal physical states of the person, a neurophysiological version of this criterion would be available. But in order to remain broadly neutral about the relationship between the mental and the physical (at least for the purposes of this paper) the concept of internality has been formulated in terms of mental states. "Mental states" is to be quite widely construed here and may be taken to include such things as thoughts, feelings, dispositions, and mental illnesses.

Easy Cases for the Externality Account of Mental Injury

The strategy that I shall adopt for introducing and assessing the externality account of *mental* injury is structurally the same as that adopted earlier for explaining and assessing the externality account of *physical* injury. First, I shall discuss cases in which the externality account appears to work relatively unproblematically. Then, I shall proceed to test the externality account against 'harder' cases: cases where it seems (at least at first sight) not to work so well.

One group of cases in which the externality account seems to work particularly well are those where individuals suffer harm as a result of being subjected to what we might call 'traumatic experiences'. Normal grief may be an example of this, since the griever is subjected to the experience of losing a loved object (normally, a person). Other, perhaps less controversial, examples might include experiencing abuse and/or violence and/or extreme danger. It seems plausible to call the mental maladies which (often) follow such experiences mental *injuries* and the reason for this is that, in each case, the main immediate cause of the malady is an external event (and the subsequent experiencing of that event) rather than some internal condition of the person.

Objection 1: Traumatic Experiences Can Cause Other Maladies

The first problem that the externality account of mental injury must face arises precisely out of these kinds of case. For although in more straightforward cases, it seems plausible to suppose that the mental maladies caused by traumatic experiences are mental injuries, this is not always the case. More specifically, it seems that traumatic experiences (especially the more severe ones) can cause conditions that we would want to call mental illness. For example, it is not uncommon for victims of torture to suffer from serious long-term mental health problems that we might be reluctant to call injuries.

There are two ways in which the externality account can deal with such cases. The first is, of course, to insist that in at least some of these cases we really are dealing with mental injury. Take the torture case for instance. Here, it does seem plausible to call many of the psychological effects of torture injuries or wounds, just as we would call many of its effects on physical health injuries or wounds. The second is to point out that injuries can themselves be the causes of other kinds of malady. For example, in the area of physical health, it is quite common for injuries (e.g. someone's leg getting damaged in a road traffic accident) to lead to complications (e.g. gangrene). Here, we would not normally say that the complications were injuries (more likely they are illness or diseases or infections) bur rather that they were caused by the (initial) injury. The same may apply to mental health. A mental injury, especially a serious one, may itself be the cause of complications which are not themselves injuries. Of course, there are difficult and interesting issues about the individuation of conditions here. In other words, how are we to distinguish an injury from its harmful effects? But leaving those aside for the present, the main point here is that injuries can themselves cause other maladies.

Hence, where a traumatic experience leads ultimately to mental illness, mental injury is normally an intermediate cause.

Objection 2: Traumatic Experiences need not be of External Events

The next objection to the externality account consists of pointing out that a traumatic experience could lead to mental injury without that traumatic experience being an experience of an *external* event, since the experience could be an hallucination or illusion.

Imagine for instance the following scenario. There are two persons, A and B, suffering from (in at least most respects) identical mental maladies - Ma and Mb respectively. Ma and Mb were each the result of traumatic experiences: Ea and Eb. Ea and Eb were, for all practical purposes, exactly qualitatively similar: i.e. indistinguishable from the perspective of the person having the experience. However, there was the following difference between Ea and Eb. Whereas Ea was a *veridical* experience (say, of real abuse) Eb was an hallucination.

Such a case would raise the following objection to the externality account. It seems as if the externality account is committed to saying that Ma *is* a mental injury (because its cause is appropriately external) whereas Mb is *not*. And this seems implausible, arbitrary and unmotivated, given that Ma is so similar to Mb.

There is, however, a reasonably straightforward way in which the externality account can deal with such cases. What matters for the purposes of the distinction between mental injury and other kinds of mental malady in these cases is the nature of the *cause* of the traumatic experience. In particular, is it external (not a mental state of the person in question) or internal (a mental state of the person in question)? Whether Mb is a mental injury, therefore, depends not on whether the apparent event experienced in Eb really took place, but rather on whether the cause of Eb was itself one of B's mental states.

There are, then, two possibilities. The first is that Eb, although a hallucination, was caused by an external event: for example, a blow to the head. If this is the case, then although Eb is indeed not an experience of something external, its cause (and therefore the cause of Mb) is external and Mb gets classified as a mental injury after all. The second is that Eb is caused by some mental event or state within B.

Here, Mb does not get classified as an injury. However, this does not seem an unreasonable classification. For if, for example, Eb was caused by some pre-existing mental condition of B (e.g. a mental illness) then it seems right to classify Mb not as a separate mental injury but rather as a symptom of the condition which caused it. And this seems right even given the superficial similarities between Ea and Eb.

The externality account then, can not only cope with this objection but seems also to make a subtle and useful distinction between Ma and Mb, by taking into account not only their experienced natures, but also their aetiology.

Objection 3: Too Many Injuries?

The third and final objection to the externality account of mental injury is that, if it is accepted, then too many ordinary mental states would get classified as injuries, thereby trivialising the concept of mental injury and making of little practical or theoretical value.

This is perhaps more of an objection to the general conception of "malady" which underpins the account of mental injury, rather than to the proposed distinction between mental injury and other maladies. The worry is that if we allow that each time someone suffers a relevant "evil" (but especially pain and loss of pleasure) as a result of a negative experience then they are mentally injured, then most of us will end up suffering from mental injuries on a more or less daily basis, since most of us frequently have experiences which cause some level of pain, or even more commonly loss of pleasure. Am I for instance mentally injured when my friend fails to turn up for a night out (loss of pleasure) or when I have my regular appointment at the dentist (minor mental distress)?

There are at least two different ways of dealing with this concern.

The first is what I term *the multiple minor maladies view*. This involves simply admitting that there are indeed vast numbers of mental injuries including the kinds of case suggested above, but to point out (a) that this is hardly surprising given that the relevant evils are matters of degree, and (b) that we are reasonably happy to accept a multiple minor maladies view of physical health. For instance, accepting that a tiny (but slightly painful) cut to the finger is an injury, albeit a trivial one seems undisturbing in the context of talk about physical health.

The second is what I term the *threshold view*. According to this, one has to suffer more than a certain amount of the relevant evils in order to be suffering from a malady at all. The obvious advantage of this view is that it exclude from the category malady and hence from the category injury a whole range of very trivial conditions. But the obvious disadvantage is that setting a quantitative threshold may lead to accusations of arbitrariness.

Conclusion

The preceding exploration has gone some way towards establishing that "mental injury" is potentially a useful concept, that it is best understood by comparing it to the concept of physical injury, and the both mental and physical injury are best defined in terms of the "externality" of their immediate causes.

References

Clouser, K., Culver, C., and Gert, B. (1997). 'Malady'. In Humber, J. and Almeder, R., eds. (1997). *What is Disease?*. Totowa, New Jersey: Humana Press.

Culver, C. and Gert, B. (1982). *Philosophy in Medicine*. Oxford: Oxford University Press.

Flew, A. (1981).Disease and Mental Disease. In Caplan, A., Engelhardt, H., and McCartney, J., eds. (1981). *Concepts of Health and Disease*. Reading, MA: Addison-Wesley.

Reznek, L. (1987). *The Nature of Disease*. London: Routledge.

Wilkinson, S. (1997) "Is grief a mental malady?", unpublished manuscript.

7 Dynamics as a Unifying Concept in Psychotherapeutic Psychiatry

An Annotation

JEREMY HOLMES

Introduction

Psychiatry traditionally divides itself into three camps - the biological, the social, and the dynamic - each with its own models of mental illness, treatment methods, and spheres of influence. There are signs that this comfortable tripartite arrangement is nearing an end. Strange portents are to be seen. Psychoanalysts feel the need to educate themselves about brain chemistry and PET scans (Olds & Cooper 1997). Evolutionary psychiatry maintains that experience and its associated behaviour are no less 'biolcgical' than are neurotransmitters (Stevens & Price 1996). Neuropharmacologists study the mechanisms by which trauma can affect brain chemistry (Nadel & Jacobs 1996) but advocate psychotherapy as, on occasion, the best treatment for depression.

Where does this leave the term dynamic in psychiatry? In this chapter I argue that despite the huge advances in brain science, contemporary psychiatry remains no less in need of the notion of psychodynamics than it was a century ago. I suggest further that the idea of psycho-dynamic psychiatry is much broader than the purely psychoanalytic, and that psychodynamics is a unifying concept for all the psychotherapies and psychological treatments. What follows is an attempt to define some key features of the dynamic perspective in psychiatry, in the hope that they may be clarified by further debate within the profession.

Although the terms *psychodynamic* and *pycho-analytic* are often used interchangeably, historically the idea of psychodynamics predates psychoanalysis. According to Ellenberger (1970) dynamic psychiatry was gradually elaborated through the course of the 19th Century, deriving originally from Leibitz' distinction between static and dynamic mechanics. Dynamic psychiatry is an Anglo-French concept elaborated among others by Brown-Sequard, Janet, and Hughlings Jackson:

> It designated the physiological aspect in contrast to the anatomic, the functional in contrast to the organic, the regressive in contrast to the status quo, and it expressed at the same time the energetic aspect, even including at times the connotation of conflict and resistance. (Elleberger 1970, p. 292)

Freud took Leibnitz' metaphor, deepening and extending it by linking it with the unconscious which he saw as 'dynamic' in the sense that it represents not just thoughts and emotions that happen to be out of awareness (i.e. in psychoanalytic terminology 'preconscious'), but those that have 'a certain dynamic character' and are actively kept apart from consciousness in spite of their intensity and activity (Freud 1912 p.434).

For Freud the dynamic nature of the psyche was particularly evident in two kinds of clinical phenomena. First was the problem of resistance in which patients fail to respond to therapy despite good rational for doing so, suggesting a part of the mind actively opposed to change, often preferring to cling to maladaptive ways of behaviour rather than relinquish the perverse satisfactions of destructiveness or a sick role. Equally convincing for Freud was the nature of memory and forgetting, especially when faced with trauma, leading him to postulate an active (and hence dynamic) banishment or repression of painful memories from consciousness.

Further evidence of the dynamic nature of the psyche came from the observation that these repressed or partially repressed memories of painful experiences, appear to influence behaviour and to produce symptoms. The continuing contemporary relevance of the dynamic concepts of resistance and repression are to be found, for example, in the accumulating evidence of high relapse rates following brief psychotherapy (Roth & Fonagy 1996), and the current debate about so-called false memory (Van de Kolk & Fisler 1996).

1. *Dynamic versus categorical approaches.* The relative success of contemporary psychiatry rests in part on its ability to define psychiatric diagnoses, and to devise specific treatments for them. The DSM and ICD have become holy writ worshipped by researchers, clinicians, and purchasers alike. They are indispensable - and yet most practising psychiatrists would concede that a purely categorical approach to psychiatry has great limitations (Hughes 1997). To claim that a particular individual suffers from schizophrenia or manic-depression gives some useful information about which drugs are likely to be effective, and in general what psychotherapeutic strategies might or might not be helpful (analytic psychotherapy: unlikely to be of benefit in schizophrenia, may have a place in resistant depression; family intervention will reduce EE and relapse in schizophrenia; cognitive therapy may be useful for delusions in schizophrenia, and may also help with drug compliance in manic-depression (Roth & Fonagy 1996) - but in the end the dynamics of a particular individual's biography and social circumstances will be the key determinants of outcome and the health resources he or she is likely to consume. Thus, for example, it has been repeatedly established that patients with coexisting personality disorder respond much less well to antidepressant therapy than those with uncomplicated depression (Sullivan et al 1994).

The multiaxial structure of the DSM and the notion of 'co-morbidity' try to capture the ways in which different diagnostic categories may coexist with an individual, but tells us little about their inter-relations. Few patients admitted to psychiatric units in the 1990s have a single diagnosis, and personality disorder researchers use the total number of personality disorders an individual is assigned as an index or severity. Something has been lost in this quest for ever-more specific and minute categories. The unity and uniqueness of the individual, and the interplay between the components that make up a personality and its vulnerabilities is the province of a dynamic psychiatry.

Of course psychodynamics needs and uses categories as well: Freud's developmental 'fixation points' or the difference between oedipal and pre-oedipal difficulties; Klein's distinction between paranoid-schizoid and depressive 'positions'; Bowlby's secure/insecure attachment dichotomy; the contrast between assumption and schema-focused work in CBT; or Minuchin's enmeshed and disorganised polarities of family functioning. What is different perhaps is that these are seen as relatively fluid and provisional - a convenient shorthand with which to focus thinking rather than static and immutable phenomena akin to medical diagnoses.

Any useful model of the mind must address not just categories but the dynamic interplay between them. There are hints in current neurobiological research that the brain itself operates in a dynamic rather than a categorical way, in the sense that *patterns* of activity rather than distinct areas of functioning underlie consciousness. Stern's (1985) dynamic notion of cross-modal 'vitality affects' which contribute to a nascent sense of self in the first year of life are based on the parent's capacity to attune to a child's rhythms and to help integrate different sensory modalities through responsive play (Hughes 1997). A similar process may be at work in the interplay of vocal tone, timbre, volume, and the pattern of turn-taking between patient and therapist in a psychotherapeutic dialogue (Holmes 1996).

2. *Defence mechanisms*. The immune system enables organisms to maintain their integrity while constantly interacting with a potentially hostile environment. Psychological defences are similarly essential if the psyche is to interact with others in a coherent and integrated way. Anxiety signals threat and is protective in the face of real or imagined danger. The concept of defence is essentially dynamic in that it postulates a balance of psychological forces in which excessive anxiety is kept in check by such strategies as obsessionality, projection, or in extreme circumstances, dissociation. Just as the immune system is overactive in atopy, so in neurotic disorders such as OCD or phobias, psychological defences can be conceptualised as disproportionate responses to the threat posed by new situations.

For Freud defences were essentially intrapsychic: a compromise between instinctual demands and the requirements and limits imposed by society. Hysteria represented the expression of sexuality in the face of social repression internalised as the superego. By contrast, a contemporary psychoanalytic perspectives see defences in interactive terms. People are programmed to seek proximity to attachment figures. If these are perceived to be hostile or unreliable, defensive strategies such as avoidance will be activated in which the individual will try to maintain contact-at-a-distance, or alternatively, in the enmeshed or preoccupied strategy to cling to their unreliable but indispensable source of security (Holmes 1996). Such patterns are readily observed on psychiatric wards. Patients suffering with Borderline Personality Disorder often appear to be attached to chaos, and become profoundly depressed when the endless dramas of their lives subside and they are faced with loneliness (Gunderson 1996).

The idea of defence implies strategies designed to avoid painful affect (Bateman & Holmes 1995). The notion of the 'manic defence' in Bipolar Disorder - a concept which originates in Kleinian psychoanalysis - provides some explanation for the common clinical observation that mania and depression may coexist; when manic patients escape momentarily from their manic flight, tears and misery often come to the surface. Similarly the dissociative phenomena that are sometimes found in extreme post-traumatic stress syndromes can be seen as defences, a response of the dynamic psyche to overwhelming stress and an attempt to protect the mind from disintegration.

The recent revival of interest in the psychological mechanisms underlying delusions and other psychotic phenomena suggest that these too can be seen as part of a defensive dynamic. Delusion-formation can be understood as an attempt to make sense of the psychic disintegration that is characteristic of psychosis (Roberts 1992). As Freud put it: "a delusion is found applied like a patch over the place where originally a rent had appeared in the ego's relation to the external world" (Freud 1924; p. 215). Current cognitive behavioural strategies in psychosis encourage the sufferer to see his psychosis in a dynamic fashion - to argue with or ignore voices, to question delusions or to see them as meaningful attempts to cope with unhappiness, or to view grandiosity as a compensation for rejection and isolation (Kingdon & Turkington 1994).

This approach to defence provides a good illustration of the interplay between categorical and dynamic thinking. Anna Freud listed at least 14 categories of defences. Contemporary psychoanalysts emphasise the spectrum from 'primitive' mechanisms such as splitting and projection, through intermediate forms such as denial and intellectualisation, to 'mature' defences such as humour and sublimation. An aim of psychotherapy would be to help shift the dynamic balance of forces from primitive to more mature defensive styles, even if the potential for regression in the face of stress is never fully transcended (Bateman & Holmes 1995). This kind of model fits well with many of the chronic and relapsing disorders that are the stuff of contemporary psychiatry.

3. *Narrative and meaning.* In common sense psychology the attribution of meaning to affective experience is essentially dynamic. 'John felt sad *because* his dog had died', 'Sally was angry *because* John had forgotten their wedding anniversary'. Psychodynamic psychiatry similarly attempts to make causal links between present experience and unconscious presumed antecedent factors. Thus denigratory auditory hallucinations in a woman who in childhood was sexually abused by her step-father might represent (a) a split off echo of the abuser's belittling and bullying attempt to force his victim to keep his secret, or (b) a manifestation of her 'survivor guilt' (however unwarranted) and so (c) an attempt to make sense of such a disastrous failure of care-giving.

In medicine generally a story, or narrative, is offered to the patient which helps to make sense of his or her distress. In dynamic psychiatry this narrative is always related to the individual life history, and is teleogical (and so dynamic) in the sense that the manifestations of illness are seen as arising out of previous experience. Equally, biological psychiatry offers a story in which an illness - whose precise origins are unknown, but presumed to be genetic, infective, or biochemical in origin - has come to afflict the sufferer. Treatment may be handled in static or dynamic mode. There is a significant difference between saying, "You have got major depression - take these pills and all will be well", and cognitive strategies along the lines of: "Your depression makes you feel guilty and responsible for your illness and that you ought to be able to overcome it, but in reality you have no more reason to hold yourself responsible for your misery than you would be if you had a broken leg or pneumonia".

Jerome Bruner (1986) argues that narrative and scientific argument are distinct approaches to the truth:

> A good story and a well-formed argument are different natural kinds. Both can be used as a means for convincing another. Yet what they convince of is fundamentally different: arguments convince of their truth, stories of their lifelikeness. The one verifies by eventual appeal to procedures for establishing formal and empirical truth. The other establishes its truth by verisimilitude. (Bruner 1986, p. 7)

As an advocate of narrative, Bruner's use of the word 'verisimilitude' is risky, given its OED definition of 'having the *appearance* of being real or true'. Critics of dynamic psychiatry might argue that this is a concession that the stories elaborated in psychotherapy can lay no more claim to the truth than can myths or fairy stories, a good example of their being the belief, widely held until trisomy was identified in 1956, that Downs Syndrome was caused by trauma in pregnancy. How can this charge be answered?

One answer is that there *is* truth in myths and fairy stories - emotional truth rather than factual truth, which can be judged, not by scientific standards, but by such tests as whether the story rings true, feels 'right', is satisfying, coherent, or touches the listener emotionally. Psychodynamic case histories are Brunerian 'good stories' which have a paradigmatic value in their own right, even though the standards of a 'well formed argument' by themselves they prove nothing. The self, it can be argued, is inherently an autobiographical or storied self, and since communication involves two or more such selves, it necessarily takes a narrative form. The criteria of a 'good story' certainly apply to psychotherapy. The dynamic psychiatrist is constantly using her intuition to evaluate a patient's narrative, asking herself if it makes sense or hangs together, questioning aspects that don't quite fit, probing cliched or phrases and well-worn narratives for what might lie beneath. The quest is always for a more elaborated, all-embracing, spontaneous, individualised, flexible story that encompasses a greater range of experience. Some patients cling to stereotyped versions of their illness, and need the irruption of free association (which is inherently 'anti-narrative'), while others , who appear to be drowning in their stories, need an injection of narrative structure and coherence (Holmes 1996).

The key focus here is not so much on experience itself, but on the *representation* of experience - the story an individual tells themselves about what has happened to them. There is evidence that the capacity for healthy representation, or Reflexive Self Function, can act as a buffer against pathological environmental experience and protect against breakdown (Fonagy et al 1995). This perspective is fundamental to cognitive strategies, whose practitioners are fond of quoting Epictetus: 'Men are troubled not so much by things, as by their appreciation of things'. Life events studies in depression have moved from looking at external factors leading to depression - early loss of mother, lack of a job, etc. - to internal or dynamic factors such as levels of mastery, a sense of being able to control one's environment and so on; similar findings are emerging in eating disorders research (Troop & Treasure 1997).

Can there also be a science of narrative, including one which would encompass the narrative aspects of psychotherapy? A useful contrast here is between metaphor and model. The dynamic unconscious is best described by imagery and metaphor, and psychodynamics relies on metaphor as a powerful way of communicating with the patient - to give just one example Rosenfeld's (1987) potent image of the 'mafia gang' which can take over the personality in borderline patients, leading to perversity and self-destructiveness. But a metaphor is not the same as a robust model (which may nevertheless originate in the mind of the researcher as an image or metaphor) which can be subjected to scientific disconfirmation.

One response is to concede that the quest for a science of psychodynamics *is* fruitless. The hermeneutic school of psychoanalysis argues that what matters in psychotherapy is not objective or 'historical' truth - which is, in their view, inherently unknowable - but 'narrative truth'. Narrative truth here refers primarily to the contemporary relationship between therapist and patient. This can be judged by the criteria mentioned on intuition, 'aesthetic' responsiveness and so on. Any connection between this present construction and past experience must necessarily be tentative and hypothetical, since we cannot know for such what *really* went on in the patient's mind as a child.

The main drawback of this position is the implication that a psychotherapeutic narrative is no more or less likely to be true than any other account of the patient's distress, whether religious, narrowly 'organic' in the psychiatric sense, or delusional. The hermeneutic turn in psychotherapy threatens to cut psychotherapy off from aspects of science - especially from evolutionary biology and developmental psychology - where dialogue between static and dynamic approaches is both necessary and possible. A more reasonable position might be to concede that while narrative truths will never have the status of the laws of physics, nevertheless there are recognised criteria by which they can be evaluated. These would include such factors as internal consistency, correspondence with established knowledge about developmental process and evolutionary biology, as well as 'aesthetic' criteria such as 'rightness' already mentioned.

Each psychodynamic school has its own vision of infancy. Some emphasise the primacy of the environment and tend to see the newborn as a tabula rasa. Others focus on the inherent programming of the infant to form attachments, and to experience extremes of emotion such as longing and hatred, and on the defences that maintain the integrity of the organism in the face of such powerful emotions. Erickson's (1968) dichotomous model sees alternative healthy or pathological developmental pathways such as trust/mistrust;industry/inferiority; generativity/stagnation; integrity/despair arising partly out of environmental influence, but also as an existential response of individuals to their fate.

Current attachment-influenced research is beginning to put some of these models to the test (Goldberg, Muir & Kerr 1995). There is convincing evidence that patterns of insecure of insecure attachment are predictable even before birth depending on parental attachment history, and by influencing the representation of experience, continue to organise an individual's relationship to the world as development proceeds. Longitudinal studies suggest links between the narrative dynamics as revealed at interview in adult life - the way people talk about themselves and their experiences - and whether they have been securely or insecurely attached as infants (Fonagy et al 1995; Holmes 1996). These kinds of findings suggest, however tentatively, that narrative *can* be subjected to scientific scrutiny, so long as science is subtle enough to encompass the complexities of dynamic and interactional psychology.

4. *The therapeutic relationship: transference and countertransference.* Social psychiatry speaks of 'treatment packages' which are 'delivered' to meet the needs of suffering clients. Some unfortunately show 'poor compliance'. A central theme of psychotherapy is the dynamic relationship between patient and therapist, which comprises conscious and unconscious contributions from both parties. Effective therapists and therapeutic teams have to be able both to participate fully with their patients while at the same time, through self-scrutiny, being aware of the dynamic interplay of which they are a part. This capacity for insight (akin to Reflexive Self Function) appears to be associated with psychological health (Fonagy et al 1995), and its enhancement is a goal of both dynamic psychotherapy and cognitive therapy.

Dynamic psychiatry can offer an understanding of how therapist or patient may sabotage the treatment alliance, the bedrock of effective therapy, whether biological or psychological. Thus, for example, Morgan's notion of the dangers of 'malignant alienation' (Watts & Morgan 1994) between staff and a suicidal patient is a dynamic concept that contrasts with a purely checklist approach to risk management. Similarly Main's (1957) classic account of staff splitting in the face of destructive borderline patients contains lessons which are rediscovered by each new generation of psychiatrists. Using an attachment framework, Dozier, Cue & Barnett (1994) have recently shown how the dynamic interplay between attachment style of mental health worker and patient may influence outcome in long-term mental illness. Insecurely attached workers tend to amplify their patient's dysfunctional attachment patterns, so that interventions with avoidant clients are shallow, but with preoccupied clients are over-involved. By contrast, securely attached workers produce a counter-balancing effect (deep interventions with avoidants, more structured with the preoccupied), which has a redressing rather than reinforcing effect on their client's difficulties.

5. *A systemic perspective.* Dynamic psychiatry is contextual and 'deconstructive' in the sense that the naive idea of illness, the role of the doctor as a benign figure, or the conscious aims of therapy are not taken at face value, but seen in a wider context of the unconscious as well as the conscious mind. Overt goals are seen as part of a psychological system

which includes drives or destructive forces of which the protagonists may be unaware.

By contrast, 'systems theory', with its emphasis on the influence of the *current* social network rather than childhood experience as a determinant of illness, originally proposed itself as an alternative to the psychoanalytic perspective (Bateson 1973). But systems theory is dynamic in that it sees the individual and her difficulties as a dynamic resultant of family forces. The commonplace observation in psychiatry, for example, that "it is not the patient but the mother (or the husband or the grandmother) who is the problem" is an example of an everyday systemic perspective which places the patient and his illness in a dynamic context of interpersonal interaction - although the risk of scapegoating needs to be taken into account. It is generally acknowledged that good practice in psychiatry requires involvement of caregivers and relatives, but without systemic understanding this can lead the therapist to become part of a malfunctioning system - taking sides with a rebellious adolescent against his parents, or being over-sympathetic to the caregiver for example - rather than a force for change.

Conclusion

These notes have perhaps done no more than state the obvious and often repeated point that the enthusiasm and undoubted success of biological approaches needs to be tempered with a balancing dynamic perspective, and to argue that this should be integral to practice, teaching and research in psychiatry. It seems that psychiatry itself, like its individual practitioners, requires reminding of psychodynamics at regular intervals (Freud advocated a re-analysis every five years for practising psychoanalysts!).

I have suggested that the idea of a dynamic psychiatry in its contemporary form encompasses not just psychoanalytic approaches, but all the major psychotherapies, including cognitive-behavioural and systemic approaches. Non-biological treatments in psychiatry are often referred to as 'psychosocial' interventions. This term - like 'psychodynamic' also a linguistic hybrid - has the advantage of being descriptive rather than theory-laden, but perhaps misses the essential features of dynamic psychiatry: an emphasis on narrative, pattern, fluidity, intuition, balance and energy. Psychoanalysis firmly established a framework for dynamic psychiatry at the turn of the previous century. These notes have tried to point to the conceptual richness of the psychodynamic approach and its potential contribution to an emerging synthesis that will form the basis for the psychiatry of the 21st century.

Acknowledgments: I am grateful to my colleague Dr Patricia Hughes for her stimulating lecture (Hughes 1997) and subsequent discussion which have contributed greatly to the evolution of this paper, and also to Anthony Bateman for helpful comments.

References

Bateman, A. & Holmes, J. (1995) *Introduction to Psychoanalysis: Contemporary Theory and Practice.* London: Routledge.

Bateson, G. (1973) *Steps Towards* and *Ecology of Mind.* London: Paladin.

Bruner, J. (1986) *Actual Minds: Possible Worlds.* Cambridge Mass: Harvard University Press.

Cooper, A. & Olds, D. (1997) Dialogues with other sciences: opportunities for mutual gain. *International Journal of Psychoanalysis*, **78**, 219-226.

Dozier, M., Cue, K. & Barnett, L. (1994) Clinicians as Caregivers: Role of Attachment Organisation in Treatment. *Journal of Consulting and Clinical Psychology*, **62**, 793-800.

Ellenberger, H. (1970) *The Discovery of the Unconscious: The History and Evolution of Dynamic Psychiatry.* New York: Basic Books.

Erikson, E. (1968) *Identity, Youth and Crisis.* New York: Norton.

Fonagy, P., Steele, M., Steele, H. et al. (1995) Attachment, the Reflective Self, and Borderline States. In *Attachment Theory: Social Developmental and Clinical Perspectives.* Eds. S. Goldberg, R. Muir & J. Kerr. New York: Analytic Press.

Freud, S. (1912) A note on the Unconscious in Psycho-Analysis. *S.E.* **12**, 262-273.

Freud, S. (1924) Neurosis and Psychosis. *S.E.* 19, 203-227.

Goldberg, S., Muir, R., & Kerr, J. (1995) *Attachment Theory: Social, Developmental and Clinical Perspectives.* New York: Analytic Press.

Gunderson, J. (1996) The Borderline Patient's intolerance of aloneness: insecure attachments and therapist availabilty. *American Journal of Psychiatry* **153**, 752-758.

Holmes, J. (1996) *Attachment, Autonomy, Intimacy: Using Attachment Theory in Adult Psychotherapy.* New York: Jason Aronson.

Hughes, P. (1997) Is the juice worth the squeeze? Psychoanalytic ideas in contemporary psychiatry. Lecture given at the Psychotherapy Section of the Royal College of Psychiatrists' Annual Meeting, Bristol.

Kingdon, D. & Turkington, D. (1994) *Cognitive Behaviour Therapy of Schizophrenia.* Hove: Laurence Erlbaum.

Main, T. (1957) The ailment. *British Journal of Medical Psychology* **30**, 129-145.

Nadel, L. & Jacobs, W. (1996) The role of the hippocampus in PTSD, panic and phobia. In *The Hippocampus: Functions and Clinical Relevance.* Ed. N. Kato. Amsterdam: Elsevier Science.

Roberts, G. (1992) The Origins of Delusion. *British Journal of Psychiatry,* **161**, 298-308.

Rosenfelt, H. (1987) *Impasse and Interpretation.* London: Routledge.

Roth, A. & Fonagy, P. (1996) *What works for Whom?* London: Guilford.

Stern, D. (1985) *The Interpersonal World of the Infant.* London: Basic Books.

Stevens, A. & Price, J. (1996) *Evolutionary Psychiatry.* London: Routledge.

Sullivan, P., Joyce & Mulder, R. (1994) Borderline Personality Disorder in Major Depression. *Journal of Nervous and Mental Disease;* **182**, 508-516.

Troop, N. & Treasure, J. (1997) Setting the scene for eating disorders, 11. Childhood helplessness and mastery. *Psychological Medicine;* **27**, 531-538.

Van de Kolk, B. & Fisler, R. (1996) Dissociation and the fragmentary nature of traumatic memories: overview. *British Journal of Psychotherapy;* **12**, 352-361.

Watts, D. & Morgan, G. (1994) Malignant alienation. *British Journal of Psychiatry;* **164**, 11-15.

8 Personal Identity and the Social Institution

R.D. (BOB) HINSHELWOOD

Introduction

The notion of personal identity was originally a useful one in trying to make sense of the work I do as a psycho-analyst. However, my sense is that in using the notion of personal identity in the field of abnormal psychology, it has become changed under my very eyes as it has dissolved and reformed itself in various ways. My understanding of the issues in philosophy about the integrity or divisibility of personal identity has been a profoundly important help to me. But in return it seems to me that abnormal psychology (especially psycho-analysis – Hinshelwood 1995, 1997 a and b) has important things to contribute to the philosophical notion. There is, in short, a reciprocal influence. One implication is that philosophy, in being applied, becomes tainted by the field it is applied to.

I shall take personal identity as a subjective experience of the individual – the answer to the question: Who or what do I believe I am?

Posing the question in this way leaves a 'gap' between 'who I experience myself to be', and who I am in some other, say objective, sense – the latter could be 'who you think I am'. For the purposes of this paper I shall call it the interpersonal definition.

Although I start with a subjective definition, I shall not exclude the other perspective. Consequently, this chapter is written in the context of an 'interpersonal' perspective. So, it will hover somewhere in this gap between the subjective and the interpersonal.

Take for example the following behaviour:

Having come together, at this appointed time, the lights dim, the curtains part and a dramatised action ensues over the course of a couple of hours, often violent, suffering or tragic. During this time the audience behave much the same, seated, calm and with a riveted attention on the figures enacting human relationships and human dilemmas on the stage. Whilst externally each member of the audience appears inactive though attentive, that attention betrays a complex and intense internal activity within themselves. One can only call it a form of identifying. The person in the audience opens himself to imagining the experiences of a figure on the stage. That figure explicitly conveys in gesture grimace and above all words, the nature of the experience for the persons in the audience to identify with. Those observing persons actually have an experience of the displayed relationships, dilemmas, humour etc. Their emotional states are co-ordinated by the action of the play; tragedy brings out sadness across the audience, humour brings out laughter, and so on.

Of course there must be some individual variation between people, but the striking quality is the identicalness of their behaviour and their internal reactions. And afterwards the persons are left with an enduring state of mind, emotional states. They also work over intelligently the experiences and emotions they have been led through. Once again, like the destructive mobs, people have voluntarily given up a degree of their individuality and entered a collective experience, knowingly and obviously with great anticipation, often with the feeling of being in the presence of something magnificent, something quite out of the ordinary. It may take a while for people to regain themselves afterwards, to disengage from feeling for the figures on the stage, to return to their own pre-occupations, to the dramas and dilemmas of their own relationships which they live in real life.

The orderliness, calmness, the dimmed lights, the comfortable surroundings, the archetected ambience and so on, are all cultivated features that allow for the intensity of group behaviour and personal identity to be orchestrated in a controlled way For a time, during the performance and until he recovers himself, the person has not quite been himself. Who, then, has he been? Perhaps he is the author of the play who has directed the sequence of experiences the person suffered; perhaps the character(s) in the play, for whom the person felt, during and after the performance. But is it possible to answer the question at all in this way? Looking in from outside the theatre as we have been doing, he is part of a group mentality. Though he may be aware of himself having the experiences, the person does suspend his awareness of himself; and no longer has his *own* pre-occupations. He gives up something of his identity in favour of having the pre-occupations that all the assembled crowd have. His identity is, in an important sense therefore, the group itself, the crowd he sits down with.

I have introduced a notion that the experience of 'who I believe I am' is connected with a process of 'identification'. In this illustration, a person identifies in various ways. Firstly with the crowd gathering, then with a person that in a couple, then with a character, or characters in the play.

Although the sense of personal identity is not the process of identification, it is an experience *formed from* that process.

Being a process, identification is a sequence of different moments. Thus the experience of being 'who I believe I am' changes with time. Thus personal identity – 'who I believe I am' - is a sequence of experiences of who I am that continue through time.

I can add that in listening to a lecturer, you are - or some of you - having my thoughts. Though you may, I hope, develop your own thoughts about mine, you have to be open first of all to have my thoughts. In this sense there is a process of identification with me, or at least an identification with my thinking, going on.

I am distinguishing the *experience* of personal identity from the interpersonal *process* of identification. Let me consider another illustration:

Consider now, being in a restaurant, near to a table with a number of people; perhaps sitting right next to them, but not part of them. They are strangers. They are however animated and merry, and with a great deal of lively talk and humour. You may overhear some of the jokes, and listen to the guffaws of uncontrollable laughter at the table. You might see the joke, know it is funny, even smile to yourself and remember to tell it the next time you are in a party like the one you are next to. But you don't guffaw with the people at the next table. You have to make overtures, smile at them, ask them a question or two, before you can find yourself invited in, and only then infected with their spirit of good-humour and laughter. Only then may you feel overwhelmed with their emotion, as they are.

However, until that moment of entry to their group, there is a boundary to the emotional infection. The laughter comes right up to you and bounces back from the edge of the group so that outside it you are only slightly moved emotionally. You can only recognise that humour is happening there, but you are not a part of it. And outside of the boundary there can be great feelings of exclusion, often hard to bear.

The experiences one has of oneself are considerably influenced by one's position *interpersonally* - within or without a group (Hinshelwood 1997a). Identification with others in this way affects, or even determines, one's own feelings, moods, and dispositions which one experiences as one's own.

The distinction between personal identity and the process of identification, and the relations between these two distinct entities, are refined especially within the field of abnormal psychology. In my own instance, I have worked this out in terms of psycho-analytic ideas and practice. The particular *processes* that go on between analyst and analysand are deeply formative of experiences (and in fact the experience of personal identity) on both sides. The processes encountered in the psycho-analytic session are called the transference and counter-transference (Sandler, Dare and Holder 1973, Laplanche and Pontalis 1980). At its very crudest one individual becomes shall we say a 'father' for the other. Experiences that might be called 'fatherly' are actually traded between the partners. I don't propose here to go into those processes in the psycho-analytic setting and how they bear on the notion of personal identity. I have described these implications elsewhere (Hinshelwood 1995, 1997b). Instead I wish to stick to more public institutions in which people experience themselves - in which they form identifications and have their personal identity.

Institutions

I want here to consider mental health institutions, those which contain vulnerable individuals - and, one might say, individuals whose vulnerability is particularly in the area of their personal identity - who they believe they are. In this case the exposure to distortion of identity is much more permanent than that in the theatre or in a restaurant, though no less radical.

The effects of the institutions became obvious in the 1950s. It gave rise to a considerable activity in what was called "medical sociology", the most well-known exponent being Erving Goffman (1961). The origins of this were in the descriptions of institutionalisation (Martin 1955), or institutional neurosis (Barton 1959). Denis Martin described what he called institutionalisation in the large and traditional mental hospital:

> The patient has ceased to rebel against, or to question the fitness of his position in a mental hospital; he has made a more or less total surrender to the institution's life... he is co-operative. Here 'co-operative' usually implies that the patient does as he is told with a minimum of questioning or opposition. This response on the part of the patient is very different from that true co-operation essential to the success of any treatment, in which the patient strives to understand, and work with, the doctor in his efforts to cure... [The] patient, resigned and co-operative... too passive to present any problem of management, has in the process of necessity lost much of his individuality and initiative (Martin 1955, pp. 1188-90).

This comes from Martin's original description. The distortion of the personality of vulnerable people resulted from the processes inherent in the institution itself. Specific power relations are clear, defining who orders and who obeys. But the patient has lost not just power, he has lost significant aspects of himself. In this account has lost his capacity for true co-operation, has lost his *active self*, and "much of his individuality and initiative". His loss of self-determination suggests a kind of deliberateness in the way identity is stripped from such patients who are already vulnerable to 'loosing their mind'.

A rather similar description was given by Tom Main when reviewing his experiences from the 1940s in mental hospitals:

Only roles of health or illness are on offer; staff to be only healthy, knowledgeable, kind, powerful and active, and patients to be only ill, suffering, ignorant, passive, obedient and grateful. In most hospitals staff are there because they seek to care for others less able than themselves, while the patients hope to find others *more* able than themselves. The helpful and the helpless meet and put pressures on each other to act not only in realistic, but also fantastic collusion... [The] helpful will unconsciously *require* others to be helpless while the helpless will *require* others to be helpful. Staff and patients are thus inevitably to some extent creatures of each other (Main 1975 p. 61).

These descriptions are remarkable for the clarity of the description of the group relations (sometimes called inter-group relations) - i.e. relations between staff and patients. But they are also remarkable in that they describe the sifting out of personality characteristics between the two groups. What patients lose of their healthy side accumulates in the identity of the staff. And what the staff lose in terms of their more negative attributes resurfaces as passivity within patients.

The redistribution of the attributes of persons occurs between two groups: The group of patients vulnerable to losing their personalities and a group of staff who need to build themselves up in successful medical and curative careers. We can see that care is benignly intended, but it can swerve off into quite extraordinary effects - normally regarded as malign. I offer this kind of personality swapping as an example of the radical construction of personal identity within the interpersonal context. The person's experience of who they believe they are is highly determined by which side of the divide between patient and staff they inhabit.

Of course this kind of deconstruction of identity occurs within relationships between groups that involve a good deal of emotional disturbance and psychopathology. As my last illustration I want to return to an observation made on a relative 'normal' group of people. I have been interested in how these divisions of personalities occur in detail, and the following illustration describes something familiar in all institutions. It does come from a mental health institution, although it concerns only the staff side of that community. In fact it was a day hospital so that attenders were not as seriously disturbed as those in the large psychiatric asylums studied by Denis Martin and Tom Main - but nevertheless unable to work and at times became psychotic.

In this observation you will see how some 'thing gets passed around through the interpersonal network. This 'something' has psychological 'substance' - rather than physical substance.

One morning Dr A arrived in the hospital building and found that the room she normally used was occupied by Dr B, a new locum. Dr A was annoyed with the newcomer. She was unable to interrupt Dr B who was interviewing a patient, so she tackled the receptionist, Mrs C, blaming her for directing Dr B to the disputed room. Mrs C was affronted and put in a bad humour by this. It happened that Dr A's ten-year-old son, D, was away from school that day and she had brought him to the hospital. Mrs C displaced her anger, when Dr A was not present, from the mother to the son. Mrs C told him off for running around and being awkward, but he remained difficult. Mrs C then tried to gain support for her criticism of D. She complained to Miss E who was one of the clinical staff in the day hospital and therefore responsible for seeing that the behaviour of patients within the hospital remained orderly.

However, instead of asserting discipline over D, Miss E attempted to calm the situation by talking to Dr A about her son. But this was not welcome. Dr A, unknown to Miss E, was still angry about Dr B and the disputed room. Dr A did not wish to control D. So, Miss E's efforts in this direction came to nothing. Miss E tried again. This time she pursued the authority structure by informing Dr F, the Consultant with overall responsibility for the hospital. She told him that D had been annoying Mrs C. Dr F considered the problem. In his experience the most troublesome children in the hospital were those who attended the weekly 'school group' for children with severe behaviour disturbances. They constituted something of a problem for him. Dr F decided that Mrs C was really annoyed with the children of this 'school group'. He conveyed his anxieties about controlling these children to the weekly staff meeting of the whole hospital.

The staff meeting discussed this and became concerned about the impact of children in the hospital as a whole. In particular there was concern that the adult day patients were disturbed by them. It was known in the past that they were disturbed by the special group of children who were autistic (another group, quite different from the 'school group'). In the end the staff meeting resolved that Miss G, the psychotherapist in charge of the Autistic Unit, should give a talk to the adult patients about the children in her unit, with the aim of reassuring the adults about their supposed anxiety.

In the network of relationships, an emotional state commenced with Dr A and flowed through a winding course, changing character and interacting with other anxieties, until it ended up as an activity of the institution. A split off piece of experience comes adrift from one person and is projected as if it were a package, a discrete quantum of experience. In the unconscious minds of the individuals, it can be taken in and given out. Nick Manning (in a personal commmunication) suggested the term "emoton", evoking a comparison with the particles of subatomic physics, like electrons. Something very personal had changed into something institutional. A depersonalisation of one individual's experience had occurred. Change from the personal to the institutional is common; and these illustrations show how something of the person is swept away into the group or institutional activity. Its *unconscious* character leads to the familiar experience of institutions as impersonal, faceless, and depersonalising of those within it.

Conclusions

What comes back from this of the philosophical notion of personal identity? The experience of 'who I believe I am' has a surprising fluidity. This is revealed by recognising the person in his interpersonal context. There appears to be a genuine discontinuity within individuals and continuity between individuals.[1]

Personal identity has been taken out of its glass case, as a specimen in museum-like isolation. I have tried to show that the individual in isolation is an artefact, and is shorn entirely of its context which make of him a person and provides for him, through his processes of identification, a personal identity.

Personal identity is therefore problematic, and my assertions have a lot of implications for philosophical and also everyday interests. I want to make three very brief comments in conclusion.

[1] I am grateful to Bill Fulford for his succinct summary of the psychoanalytic discoveries.

1. First of all; Personal identity, what is it? Clearly personal identity has *some* connection with the sequence of experiences that are composed from the interpersonal context in which for the moment the person exists.

Though his experiences are formed from his context, we see that more than that, certain actually aspects of character are added or subtracted from him. If personal identity is something to do with a self reflection on himself, and a sense of his 'continuity of being'[2] then this has little to do with a continuity of experiences and functions. 'Who I believe I am' is much more to do with a sense of a locus in which experiences occur and at which mental functions happen. Mental events are therefore more like beads on a string.

2. The recent philosophical debates about the discreteness or otherwise of identity (Parfitt 1984, Glover 1988, Harré 1979, Braude 1995), arise from the concern to understand irrationality within an analytic philosophical tradition which starts with the Cartesian notion of the person as rational.

The idea is that self-deception and acrasia could arise from minds being divided in parts which act against each other. The metaphysical problems arising from this are severe (Gardner 1995), and some philosophers have turned to empirical data -- from neurophysiology on bisected brains (Nagel 1971), or from the psychology of multiple personalities (Braude 1995) -- now called dissociative identity disorder. Much of this is inconclusive. In particular whether there is really a condition in which a mind can actually divide into two separate active parts without recognising their links with each other.

The type of phenomena that I have reported on, discovered initially in psycho-analysis, do fill the bill for being truly divided minds.

---

[2] This phrase is borrowed from Winnicott (1960).

3. If a mind is truly divided there are profound implications for ethics and moral philosophy. For instance, Braude, in discussing multiple personalities has remarked on the odd case in which one of the 'alters' of such a person has committed a crime, do all the alters have to stand in the dock, are they all punished, or do each of the separate alters require their own legal representation?[3]

In my own work I have been interested in the professional ethics of working with divided minds. Since in medical ethics the central pivot is the autonomy of the patient, one has to ask; which part of the patient should have autonomy? Which must give informed consent? This particularly acute as a problem in psycho-analytic treatments where such splits in the person are made manifest in the course of the treatment itself.

References

Barton, R. (1959) *Institutional Neurosis*. Bristol: Wright.

Braude, S. (1995) *First Person Plural: Multiple Personality and the Philosophy of Mind.* Lanham: Rowman and Littlefield.

Gardner, S. (1995) Comment on 'Social relocation of personal identity'. *Philosophy, Psychiatry and Psychology* **2:** 209-214.

Goffman, E. (1961) *Asylums*. New York: Doubleday.

Glover, J. (1988) *I: The Philosophy and Psychology of Personal Identity.* London: Allen Lane, The Penguin Press.

Harré, R. (1979) *Social Being.* Oxford: Blackwell.

Hinshelwood, R.D. (1995) 'Social relocation of personal idsentity through splitting, projection and introjection'. *Philosophy, Psychiatry, Psychology* **2:** 185-204.

Hinshelwood R.D. (1997 a) Primitive mental processes: psycho-analysis and the ethics of integration. *Philosophy, Psychiatry, Psychology 4.*

[3] Was the psychiatrist so unreasonable for billing the insurance company in North America when, trying to treat a women with a dissociative disorder comprising 169 alters, he billed the company for group therapy for each of them!

Hinshelwood R.D. (1997b) *Therapy or Coercion: Does Psychoanalysis Differ from Brainwashing?* London: Karnac.
Laplanche and Pontalis (1980) *The Language of Psycho-Analysis*. London: The Hogarth Press.
Martin, D. (1955) Institutionalisation. *Lancet* **2:** 1188-90.
Main, T.H. (1975) Some psychodynamics of large groups. In Kreeger, Lionel (ed) *The Large Group*. London: Constable. Reprinted in Main T.H. (1989) *The Ailment*. London: Free Association Books.
Nagel, T. (1971) Bain bisection and the unity of consciousness. *Synthese 2*: 396-413. Reprinted 1979 in Thomas Nagel *Mortal Questions*. Cambridge: Cambridge University Press.
Parfit, D. (1984) *Reasons and Persons*. Oxford: Oxford University Press.
Sandler, J., Dare, C., and Holder, A. (1973) *The Patient and the Analyst*. London: George Allen and Unwin.

9 Therapeutic Jurisprudence and Psychopathy

A Philosophical Exploration

CHRISTOPHER HEGINBOTHAM

It has often been noted that mental health law has had a cyclical, or pendulum like, history (e.g. Jones, 1991). Legal formulation has tended to swing from allowing clinicians extensive discretion to act in their patients' best interests, towards detailed legal regulation and procedural controls, and back again towards discretion. Whilst the Mental Health Act 1959 was associated with extensive clinical discretion, the Mental Health Act 1983, and comparable legislation for Scotland and Northern Ireland, is associated with tighter legal regulation and greater use of legal remedies. Many more cases have been brought to the courts, under the current Act, to test the law and to seek reforms.

Meanwhile, in the United States of America, the ten years from the mid 1980s to the mid 1990s have seen a new approach to mental health law develop and flourish, known as 'therapeutic jurisprudence'. Does this represent a genuinely new departure or approach to mental health law and the relationship between psychiatrists and lawyers? What assumptions does it make about the nature of mental health, about law and change? What are its philosophical underpinnings? Is it relevant to the debate about the need for a new Mental Health Act, which has been argued? What can therapeutic jurisprudence tell us about appropriate disposal of persons with personality disorder and psychopathy?

Many would agree that 'therapeutic jurisprudence' (TJ) was, in retrospect, an unfortunate label to adopt. It implies that TJ is, or involves, a body of explicit beliefs and/or values. Of course it involves a number of assumptions, which it is important to make explicit, but it is much more appropriate to consider it as a method. "Therapeutic jurisprudence is the study of the role of the law as a therapeutic agent". (Wexler and Winick, 1996, p. xvii)

TJ is concerned with whether the law, which is perceived as a mechanism, has a therapeutic effect. It concerns the effects of the law. "Legal rules, legal procedures, and the roles of legal actors (such as lawyers and judges) constitute social forces that, like it not, often produce therapeutic or anti-therapeutic consequences". (Wexler and Winick, 1996, p. xvii) TJ examines whether the effects of a law are beneficial, that is therapeutic, and if not, whether they can be made therapeutic. "Therapeutic jurisprudence proposes that we be sensitive to those consequences, and that we ask whether the law's anti-therapeutic consequences can be reduced, and its therapeutic consequences enhanced, without subordinating due process and other justice values". (Wexler and Winick, 1996, p. xvii)

Therapeutic jurisprudence recognises that the law can help – or hinder – people with a mental disorder. It is an implicit value that the law ought to have a therapeutic effect, if that is possible, and that any anti-therapeutic effects ought to be minimised. Thus it involves both descriptive and normative analyses. TJ assists in determining the effects of the law and in finding ways of stating or using the law so that it will have a beneficial.

The word 'therapeutic' is involved because TJ, the method, was initially utilised on mental health law issues. However it has since been used on a much wider range of legal issues. For example, Wexler's and Winick's (1996) latest collection of studies includes chapters by a wide range of authors on corrections, criminal law and sentencing, family and juvenile law, sex, disability, health, personal injury, evidence, industrial relations and contract law. The term 'jurisprudence' is used because it involves a study of the law, its limits and methods. Unfortunately, when the two words are used together some people assume that TJ is a philosophy, or set of arguments, designed to justify the imposition of paternalistically determined 'therapeutic' outcomes on patients without any recognition of the value judgements involved. As has already been noted, and will be emphasised further, TJ scholars are well aware that what is 'therapeutic' cannot be assumed, either generally or for particular patients. Indeed a particular virtue of TJ studies is a readiness to question liberal assumptions about what is appropriate. (For examples see, generally, Winick, 1997.)[1]

In retrospect it does not appear too surprising that TJ developed in the late 1980s and early 1990s in the USA. The TJ opus is dominated by the contributions of lawyers, most of whom are academics, although a growing proportion are practising judges. The 'realist' approach to the study of law has always been stronger in the USA. This approach argues that what actually happens and what legal officials do, for example which laws they enforce and which in effect they ignore, is more worthy of study than that which is declared in law books and in libraries. When TJ is used to analyse legislation and Appeal Court precedents, it is done so as to discover whether the law is declared, or a procedure utilised, will have beneficial effects.[2]

Therapeutic jurisprudence may also be seen as a reaction against the perceived failure of the test-case strategy. In both the USA and the UK taking cases to the courts, about mental health law issues, has sometimes led to judgements which advance the interests of mentally disordered people. In this way the law is 'tested'. Sometimes unfortunately it has a negative effect and even if a court interprets a law in favour of patients the government can always undermine the decision by changing the law. This is even easier in the UK with the absence of a written constitution. In the USA after a more liberal period in the 1960s and 1970s, conservative judges were appointed to the Supreme Court. In both countries (and indeed in many others) government policy, in recent decades, has been dominated by reductions in public expenditure. The test case strategy has not proved a consistently productive tactic, despite occasional causes for excitement. The adoption of the European Convention of Human Rights into UK law is likely to yield some interesting results.

Like the test case strategy TJ is another means by which the perceived interests of people with mental disorders may be advanced. It is decidedly reformist, but has much more potential. It is not restricted to the kind of issues that can be placed before a court, and does not require someone to have experienced the actual problems and to be able to fund litigation. Perhaps most significantly, it is 'apolitical'. A TJ study may approve of the goals of a particular law because they are therapeutic but that study may point out that the legal means chosen to achieve those goals are ineffective or inefficient. Equally it may disapprove of the goals of a law because they are counter productive or anti-therapeutic. By focusing upon efficiency TJ complements modern political considerations. But that does not prevent TJ from being radical as it may demonstrate that extent to which a current law is inappropriate or inefficient. Therapeutic jurisprudence is not ideological, in the sense of pursuing a particular policy or set of values, beyond seeking more therapeutic outcomes for more people, both quantitatively and qualitatively.

Therapeutic jurisprudence may be seen also in small part, as a reaction against the nihilism of critical legal studies which emphasised moral relativism and which attacked arguments to the effect that *law* and legal principles had some form of greater authority independent of being *law*. Critical legal theory denies that law is above or independent of policies. "The discretionary nature of court decisions, the importance of social and political judgements, and the dominance of the ideology of advanced capitalism characterise our judicial process far better than any notions of objectivity, expertise, or science" (Kairys, 1982a, p.6).

Therapeutic jurisprudence does not pretend that the law is politically neutral, but its practitioners do not conclude, from that, that there is nothing that they can do. Rather TJ provides scholars and practitioners, who wish to improve the life experiences of people with mental disorders, with practical tools and a coherent perspective with which to advocate and justify change. Therapeutic jurisprudence thus resides within the tradition of liberal reformism, and indeed may be a product of its times. Across the developed nations, at least, there is limited public support for people with mental disorders, prisoners and similar excluded or disadvantaged groups. Direct public funding of services for disadvantaged people is being reduced. There is widespread support for policies of community support and care but inadequate funding leading to greater pressure on voluntary and extended family services. There is extensive wariness of political ideology and managerialism, although wrongly, often assumed just to be a technical skill.

Therapeutic jurisprudence is liable to be associated with utilitarianism. Laws ought to be beneficial and effective. It is the instrumental, rather than the symbolic, effect of law that matters. It is not their nature, quality or essence that matters but rather their effects.

"The greatest good of the greatest number" is *not* a core feature of TJ; the focus is not the group - for example mentally disordered people , but rather the individual. The question to ask is: is this law therapeutic for this person? Of course by happy coincidence, a law which is therapeutic for one is likely to be therapeutic for many others. Certainly it would be more efficient to have laws that produced the greatest therapeutic good for the greatest number of people but there is nothing in TJ that encourages or authorises the imposition of a non-therapeutic outcome upon an individual.

Therapeutic jurisprudence provides no support or consolation for professional paternalism. Therapeutic outcomes cannot justify trampling upon individuals' civil and other legal rights. As Wexler has written, civil rights always trump therapeutic outcomes (ref). But, equally, TJ does not take civil rights for granted. It is only too easy to turn a perceived civil right into a mantra and fail to consider its effects. For example Winick (1997) has examined the consequences of judicial declarations that someone is incapable. The United States Supreme Court, in Zinermon v. Burch (494 U.S. 113, 19xx), laid down a requirement for an assessment of competency even before patients are admitted, voluntarily, to a mental hospital. This may be seen as protecting their civil rights because the individuals may being pressurised by other people to enter hospital or their perceived disorder may be no more than eccentricity or behaviour of which some people disapprove. Such protection may be counter productive.

Winick examines the behavioural science literature, and notes, in particular, Scheff's (1974) work on labelling theory. This indicates that labelling someone in a particular way, for example as incompetent, often has the effect of the label, it makes the person incapable. He notes Seligman's (1975) work on learned helplessness to the effect that people generalise their incapacity in one area to others, presume that it is a stable state and their problem rather than the consequence of a lack of appropriate services or support. From this Winick considers the consequences, for individuals, of incompetency hearings. Someone may, at a particular stressful or unsupported time in his or her life, be incompetent, at least at making certain decisions, A judicial hearing may so decide, and support voluntary admission to hospital. But the effect of the process, with all the associations of rational argument, independence and fairness that run with judicial hearings, is liable to be that the individual comes to believe that he or she is more incapable, and on a wider range of issues, than he or she actually is. Whilst the decision-making process may have been designed to protect civil liberties by determining whether people are incapable, it is liable to have the effect of confirming people in their self-concept of incompetence and inability to change things. A judgement, which seems to uphold the importance of civil liberties, may thus remove them!

Even if an hypothesis about the likely effects of a law, such as that concerning the consequences of declaring people incapable, was confirmed by research that would not provide an automatic answer as to how the law should be amended. TJ is not an excuse for imposing that which works for most people onto everyone. The response should be that we seek methods of minimising the likelihood, or degree, of 'anti-therapeutic' effects for each individual. Mental health law, quite rightly given the issues concerned, is controversial. TJ does not deny this. TJ scholars recognise that there are difficult issues of competing values involved. The method encourages them to be 'up front' about their assumptions and values. TJ provides a valuable guard against sloppy thinking and liberal contentment.

That is not to deny that TJ has its critics. Some believe that, even if there is no explicit ideology or agenda there must be one which is implicit. For them it is sophisticated means of justifying more intervention in patients' lives, and bodies, in the name of therapy and the hegemony of psychiatry. The concern about the value-ladenness of the 'therapeutic' enterprise might be better stated as a concern with problem-solving. The motivation in TJ is to solve problems when, until the effects of a law had been reviewed there was not thought to be a problem. There is likely to be a tendency to associate the problem with the patient, and in doing so we reinforce the separateness and distinctiveness of mental disorder rather than the continuities between those with mental disorder and others.

The most perceptive criticism of TJ has come from one of its supporters. Slogobin (1996) has identified five dilemmas, although these are not unique to TJ. Rather most of them arise from empiricism, and the others flow from TJ being normative as well as analytical and descriptive. First there is the 'identity dilemma'. This highlights the problems in determining what is 'therapeutic'. Similar issues arise in any empirical work where the authors move on to suggest action. Legal scholarship, whether doctrinal or empirical, is usually associated with advocacy of change. The second dilemma concerns the nature of what is 'therapeutic' and that what it involves can vary from person to person. Whilst, for example, we generally support the maintenance and enhancement of autonomy that will not be 'therapeutic' for everyone. This reinforces the point that TJ is individualistic rather than collectivist in its analysis, and thus the 'problem' of application.

The third dilemma arises out of TJ's advocacy of empirical research to test hypotheses about the law and its actual effects. Whilst many theories can be tested empirically many others cannot. Sometimes poorer quality research will have to be undertaken because it would be unethical, possibly unlawful, to employ a control group. But this problem is certainly not limited to TJ. Fourth, empirical research may produce mixed or inconsistent results. For example, it may suggest that incompetency hearings are sometimes valuable but not always. When this occurs it challenges those who wish to make reform proposals to come up with sophisticated techniques that can take these differences into account. Finally Slogobin notes that TJ provides no answer to the problems that arise when competing values are involved. The problems will still have to be determined by a balancing of the values involved. This fifth dilemma or critique actually undermines the other criticism which suggests that TJ does have a value agenda.

Others may wish to argue, in effect, that TJ is too rational. Mental health, is a very emotional topic, both for those affected by a disorder or disability and for the public. These are not issues, the argument may run, which can or should be resolved by 'rational' means; the public will always be frightened of, and exaggerate, the risk of harm by a mentally disordered person. Fortunately that is a proposition which could, in part, be tested empirically.

Therapeutic jurisprudence is, in one sense, very tame, it is gentle, polite, rational, reformism. However it is also suggested that TJ is radical in that it, breaks critically with the past, and with the tired and unimaginative pendulum swings between laws which support clinical discretion and other laws that seek to provide extensive legal regulation. It may provide a way out of the unfruitful antagonisms between lawyers and psychiatrists. It may carry with it a number of assumptions about what is 'therapeutic' but, because it is a method rather than a doctrine, it encourages its adherents to be explicit about their assumptions.

We now turn to personality disorder and psychopathy, and consider how therapeutic jurisprudence can assist on dealing with this class of persons. Persons who display psychopathic tendencies and have deviant personality traits present a significant challenge to health and criminal justice agencies. Personality disorder ranges over a wide spectrum and is often compounded by various forms of mental illness or substance misuse, sometimes in association. A great deal of thought has been given to the proper sentencing, disposal and treatment of persons with psychopathy. Whilst a common consensus is yet to emerge changes in attitudes amongst clinicians to the possible treatability of some personality disorders, and wide ranging interest amongst relevant professional disciplines, offers an opportunity for a re-evaluation of the treatment and disposal of such persons.

Psychopathy and Personality Disorder

Personality disorder is poorly defined. A variety of instruments have been developed to measure the extent of personality disorder though it is not proved possible to define tightly the bounds of differing types of PD. Psychopathy is usually described as the most extreme form of personality disorder in which the individual lacks empathy with others and has callous indifference or unconcern for the feelings and pain of other persons. In practice psychopathy like many other personality disorders is a variable state and may be more or less amenable to treatment dependent upon the genesis of the disorder, the extent to which the individual may be motivated to achieve personal change (although one facet of psychopathy is the lack of goal directed motivation), and the attitude of the treating clinician to psychological intervention and therapy.

Persons with psychopathy are usually perceived as untreatable by normal psychiatric modalities and this perception has led to a clear cut two level distinction in treatment and disposal. At the first level persons with psychopathy usually present following some anti-social incident often but not always including harm to others. Presentations may be via the courts or directly to mental health services; but often mental health care is denied on the grounds that the disorder is untreatable and that the person cannot be detained under relevant sections of the Mental Health Act 1983. The Crime (Sentences) Act 1997 changes mechanisms of disposal and may change the behaviour of treating clinicians as there is now an expectation that mental health services will give closer consideration to the needs of this class of persons.

The second level occurs once an individual has committed an offence serious enough to warrant a custodial sentence when, occasionally in the past, and probably more frequently in the future as a result of the 1997 Act, persons with psychopathy may become patients of the mental health services. The second level is triggered once the individual commits a dangerous act or harms another. Thus the test of admission is not dangerousness per se or potential dangerousness to self or other, but the commission of a dangerous or harmful act. Many mental health professionals feel unable to act even though they view persons with psychopathy as simply 'offences waiting to happen'. There are two reasons for this: the legislative framework at best discourages and at worst disallows detention of persons for whom medical treatment (in its wider sense) is unlikely to work; and second, many such persons are felt not to be treatable especially in the timescale allowed within the review mechanisms under the Mental Health Act. The subtle change brought about by the Crime (Sentences) Act changes the test from 'treatability' to 'appropriateness of detention for treatment'. This shift may over time change behaviours in treating clinicians especially if psychological therapies (for example, cognitive behaviour therapy) begin to show some benefits in the medium to long term treatment of persons with psychopathy.

Custodial Care and Treatment

Psychopathy requires a new response (i) because such persons can be dangerous and waiting until a serious crime is committed is a poor, although understandable, public policy response in the absence of effective preventive detention, and (ii) because the response once a crime is committed is a long term custodial sentence which is neither in the interests of the individual or of society. The individual does not receive the treatment that he or she requires yet is discharged from prison some years later probably to re-offend; and the cost to society of custodial care is enormous when medium term (1,2,3 years) clinical care in secure settings may be both beneficial to the person and cost effective.

If such developments are to occur it will be necessary to define as rigorously as possible the class of persons to which such treatment applies. Because personality disorder runs along a wide spectrum and because there are other deviant categories within that spectrum (for example: paedophiles; 'ordinary' criminals) it is essential to be clear what is intended. An approach to this taxonomy is to define a number of traits or factors which apply differentially to various classes of persons with deviant personality and to examine the particular nature of psychopathy against those parameters and in comparison to other sub-groups. For our purposes here eight such factors can be defined. These are:

motivation
empathy
participant reactive attitudes
dangerousness
prudence (in decision making)
evaluation (of the decision)
forecast consequences (of decisions and actions taken)
capacity and competence.

If we were to consider each of these in turn we would see that there are overlapping elements between people with psychopathy and other deviant personalities such as paedophiles, but there are also some significant differences. By and large people with psychopathic disorder are not person centred, lack empathy to **all** classes of persons and as a result of early childhood experiences often lack self esteem. Their participant reactive attitudes are seriously impaired(see Benn, Chapter 3 above) or non existent and they are dangerous because of callous indifference or unconcern for the feelings and pain of others. They are also poor at making long term decisions and are not goal directed, but are often impulsive and concerned with some immediate gratification (such as obtaining illicit substances). Their competence in decision making is poor though as has been noted (Maher, 1990) they sometimes make good 'streetwise' decisions at the margins of their activity - for example, in evading the police.

By comparison, other deviant personalities are often motivated by specific pleasures or gratification and will make substantial efforts to both gratify those urges and to cover their tracks. Such deviant personalities may not necessarily lack self esteem and may appear reasonably empathetic except with those against whom their urges are directed. This goal directed behaviour is a crucial difference even though these are goals which society has determined are unacceptable and against which sanctions apply. Thus the key difference between persons with generalised psychopathic disorder and persons with other deviant personalities such as paedophilia is that in the former case there is little considered goal directed behaviour, whilst in the latter there is carefully considered behaviour aimed at achieving well defined goals.

It is not unreasonable therefore for society to establish and exact high penalties for those who knowingly set about achieving such goals (even though some forms of psychological treatment may eventually be found to work). Such deviant personalities are morally unattractive and naturally attract societies dis-pleasure; whilst the psychopath, although potentially dangerous, should be considered a person who is unable, for one reason or another, to manage his or her non-prudential dysfunctional relationships; in a paradoxical sense he or she **is** deserving of society's concern. How that concern is manifest is a matter for further consideration but suggests there is a fairly clearly defined category of persons for whom some special service may be needed.

The more difficult distinction is with those criminal persons who are intellectually impaired in the sense that their competence and possibly underlying capacity is reduced but who are not psychopathic in the sense of lacking empathy or participant reactive attitudes. There will be some few persons about who making a distinction may be difficult but in these cases it would not be unreasonable to err on the side of caution and if they are regular re-offenders to include them in an appropriate treatment regime.

Applying therapeutic jurisprudence to the treatment of persons with psychopathy yields interesting results. The Mental Health Act 1983 does not provide a firm foundation on which to decide the appropriate care support or treatment of persons with psychopathy. Section 2 of the Act which provides for compulsory admission and detention for up to 28 days for assessment or for assessment followed by treatment is based on the following grounds:

> the patient is suffering from mental disorder of a nature or degree which warrants such detention for a limited period, and
>
> (s/he) ought to be so detained for his (or her) own health or safety or for the protection of others.

The term 'mental disorder' is not defined yet the grounds for admission or detention for compulsory treatment for up to 6 months in Section 3 of the Act is based on the following grounds:

> the patient is suffering from mental illness, mental impairment, severe mental impairment, or psychopathic disorder. The patient is suffering from any other disorder or disability of mind cannot be detained for treatment under this order, and the mental disorder is of a nature or degree which makes it appropriate for the patient to receive such treatment in hospital, and
>
> it is necessary in the interests of his health or safety or for the protection of other that he (she) should receive such treatment and it cannot be provided unless he (she) is detained.

The Act also stipulates that for a patient suffering from psychopathic disorder it is necessary that medical treatment is likely to alleviate or prevent deterioration.

The Crime (Sentences) Act 1997 amends this situation by providing a subtle shift in the grounds for detention. This Act introduced a 'hybrid' order enabling patients to be given a prison sentence of fixed duration but that the sentence could be served in a secure mental health services setting. Preparatory work before the Act was passed had incorporated the notion of 'uncertain treatability' but this was changed by government to that of culpability, and thus punishment, implying a concern for dangerousness and public protection. The test for in-patient mental health care thus changes from one of 'treatability' to one of 'appropriateness of detention for treatment'; a change from the position that 'treatment is likely to alleviate or prevent a deterioration' as in Section 3 of the 1983 Act, to one where detention is appropriate such that treatment might be given **whether or not** the treatment is likely to be effective.

From the perspective of therapeutic jurisprudence this is a mixed result. Detaining persons against their will in mental health facilities if they do not have an evidently or readily treatable mental illness is a potentially draconian result. The alternative is to recognise that the person has committed an offence for which there is a tariff and that sentence should be served and the offender then released. However this raises two questions which challenge any disposal of persons with psychopathy:

- first, what do we mean by treatability, and can we say that any mental disorder is wholly refractory and completely untreatable?
- second, is it reasonable to set a fixed term sentence when it is likely that on release the person will re-offend? - in other words what preventive measures can and should be taken by society?

To what extent is the law as presently drawn assisting in providing a therapeutic approach to the needs of people with psychopathy? If we take the view that persons with psychopathy by definition have no empathy, no participant reactive attitudes and at all times complete callous indifference to the feelings of others, then, as Piers Benn has suggested (Chapter 3, above) that society has every right to treat the person as if they are not part of the normal web of human interaction. Conversely if persons with psychopathy range along a spectrum from those who have diminished or impaired emotional ability to interact with others to those who are wholly incapable of such interactions, then there will be some, indeed many, individuals for whom some form of appropriate intervention may be desirable.

The law needs to effect appropriate treatments for such persons without becoming shallow or romantic. In practice the legal formulation now available could be used to ensure that persons with psychopathy are detained in hospital for psychological treatment for longer periods of time which of themselves encourage the patient to enter into long term therapeutic commitments. The wording of Sections 2 and 3 of the Mental Health Act 1983 encouraged a belief in patients that review of detention would mean their stay in hospital would be a maximum of 6 months. That did not encourage patients to take a long term view of possible therapeutic relationships.

An additional feature of the Mental Health Act 1983 and the Crime (Sentences) Act 1997 is the emphasis on dangerousness. Although Section 2 and 3 of the 1983 Act talks of the patients 'health or safety or for the protection of others' the emphasis has traditionally focused on harm to self or others. Because of the 'folk' understanding of psychopathy (bad not mad), the reluctance of many mental health professionals to treat persons with psychopathy, and the dangerousness component of the grounds for compulsory admission, the ever present ambience around psychopathy is one of violence and harm, with an implied emphasis on custody rather than treatment. In certain respects therefore the shift in emphasis from 'treatability' to 'appropriateness of detention for treatment' may be therapeutically beneficial, if for no other reason then it overcomes the reluctance of some mental health professionals to enter any form of treatment regime once a patient is labelled psychopathic.

Attitudes to treatment have been changing recently as many enlightened mental health professionals recognise the value of forensic psychotherapy and psychological therapies (such as cognitive behaviour therapy), in helping persons with personality disorder and psychopathic personality. This is to be welcomed as it might be argued that psychopathy is in may senses a true mental disorder brought about by psychological stress and pressure, whereas many mental illnesses, so called are in practice the mental manifestations of possible physical diseases. Whilst we know too little about disorders such as schizophrenia and manic depression there are many physicalist theories which are not relevant to our understanding of psychopathy.

In summary, therapeutic jurisprudence is one way in which we can 'take another look' at psychopathy, providing an alternative perspective on disposal, rooted not in a traditional 'mad, bad, or sad' paradigm, but instead in a reasoned approach to responsibility and causal determinism. Psychopathy may still provide many challenges, but we should find a way to to allow the person behind the label to appear, and to offer care and support to the person rather than simplistically focussing on, and indeed incarcerating the label.

Notes

1. The principal progenitors of therapeutic jurisprudence are David Wexler, Professor of Law and Psychology at the University of Arizona (and also the University of Puerto Rico, and Professor Bruce Winick of the School of Law at the University of Miami. Both have had a substantial connection with mental health law issues. Wexler (1981) had demonstrated an empirical interest in what actually happened in mental health services, for example the quality of commitment hearings, and not just in 'doctrinal' law (the frequently sophisticated linguistic analysis of statutes and case-law precedents). Winick was Director of Court Mental Health Services in New York. Both Wexler (1990) and Winick (1997) have published collections of some of their own TJ work as well as jointly edited two collections (1991, 1996).

2. In the USA law is a postgraduate degree course and more open to inter-disciplinary studies. Indeed Wexler (1993) has identified TJ as part of a new kind of legal scholarship which emphasises the contributions of legal officials, as well as judges and legislations, and which is inter-disciplinary in character. Whilst psychology and law studies, and courses, are well developed in North America they are only beginning in the UK. (The first European psychology and law journal was founded in 1992: Law and Human Behaviour, published in the USA, began in 1977). Therapeutic jurisprudence studies regularly draw upon insights from the behavioural sciences.

"We began to understand law as a system of applied psychology. Law, after all, seeks to order human behaviour. Yet the law often seemed to misunderstand or misapply psychology." (Winick, 1997, p.10)

References

Benn P. (1998) 'Freedom, Resentment and the Psychopath', Chapter 3 above.

Crombag H.M.F. (1984) Some psychological observations on Mens Rea, (in) Psychology and Law, Muller D.J. Blackman, D.E. and Chapman A.J (eds), Chichchester: Wiley (pp. 55-66).

Dolan B. and Coid J. (1993) *Psychopathic and Anti-social Personality Disorder*, London: Gaskell.

De Girolamo G. and Reich J.H. (1993) *Personality Disorders*, Geneva, WHO.

Heginbotham C. (1996) 'Mental Disorder, Multiple Diagnosis and Secure Provision' in Tam H. ed. *Punishment, Excuses and Moral Development*, Aldershot: Avebury.

Jones K. 'Law and mental health: Sticks or carrots?' in *150 Years of British Psychiatry 1941 – 1991*, London: Gaskell (pp. 89-102).

Kairys D. (1992a), 'Introduction', in Kairys D. (ed) *The Politics of Law: A Progressive Critique*, (ed) Pantheon: New York (pp. 1-10).

Kairys D. (1992b), 'Legal reasoning', in Kairys, D. (ed) *The Politics of Law: A Progressive Critique*, Pantheon: New York (pp. 11-18).

Law Commission (1975), *Mental Incapacity* (Law Com No 231), London: HMSO.

Maher B. (1989) 'The Irrelevance of Rationality', in Spitzer, M. and Maher, B. (1989) *Philosophy and Psychopathology*, New York: Springer-Verlag.

Scheff T.J. (1974), 'The labelling theory of mental illness', *American Sociological Review*, **39**: pp.444-447.

Slogobin C. (1996), 'Therapeutic jurisprudence: Five Dilemmas to ponder', in *Therapeutic Jurisprudence Applied: Essays on Mental Health Law* (ed) Winick, B.J. Durham (N. Carolina): Carolina Academic Press.

Wexler D. B. (1981), *Mental Health Law: Major Issues*, New York: Plenum Press.

Wexler D.B. (1990), *Therapeutic Jurisprudence*, Durham (N. Carolina): Carolina Academic Press.

Wexler D.B. (1993), 'Therapeutic jurisprudence and Changing conceptions of legal scholarship', *Behavioural Sciences & Law*, 1(1): pp.17-30.

Wexler D.B. and Winick B.J. (1996), *Law in a Therapeutic Jurisprudence*, Durham (N. Carolina), Carolina Academic Press.

Winick B.J. (1997) *Therapeutic Jurisprudence Applied: Essays on Mental Health Law*, Durham, N. Carolina: Carolina Academic Press.

Winick B.J. (1997b), 'The side-effects of incompetency labelling' (in) *Therapeutic Jurisprudence Applied: Essays on Mental Health Law* (ed) Winick, B.J. Durham (N. Carolina): Carolina Academic Press.

For Product Safety Concerns and Information please contact our EU representative GPSR@taylorandfrancis.com Taylor & Francis Verlag GmbH, Kaufingerstraße 24, 80331 München, Germany

Batch number: 10725802

Printed by Printforce, the Netherlands